CLINIC CONSULT
PULMONOLOGY

Tuberculosis

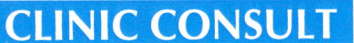
CLINIC CONSULT
PULMONOLOGY

Tuberculosis

Author

Digambar Behera MD DNB FCCP FAMS
FICP FNCCP FICS FICP FAPSR

Senior Professor and Head
Department of Pulmonary Medicine
WHO Collaborating Centre for Research and
Capacity Building in Chronic Respiratory Diseases
Postgraduate Institute of Medical Education and Research
Chandigarh, India
Former Director LRS Institute of Tuberculosis and
Respiratory Diseases (Now known as National Institute of
Tuberculosis and Respiratory Diseases)
Chairman, National Task Force for involvement of
Medical Colleges in RNTCP, Government of India;
Chairman, National Operational Research Committee,
RNTCP, Government of India

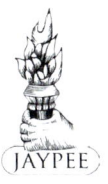

The Health Sciences Publisher

New Delhi | London | Panama

Jaypee Brothers Medical Publishers (P) Ltd

Headquarters

Jaypee Brothers Medical Publishers (P) Ltd
4838/24, Ansari Road, Daryaganj
New Delhi 110 002, India
Phone: +91-11-43574357
Fax: +91-11-43574314
Email: jaypee@jaypeebrothers.com

Overseas Offices

J.P. Medical Ltd
83 Victoria Street, London
SW1H 0HW (UK)
Phone: +44 20 3170 8910
Fax: +44 (0)20 3008 6180
Email: info@jpmedpub.com

Jaypee-Highlights Medical Publishers Inc
City of Knowledge, Bld. 237, Clayton
Panama City, Panama
Phone: +1 507-301-0496
Fax: +1 507-301-0499
Email: cservice@jphmedical.com

Jaypee Brothers Medical Publishers (P) Ltd
17/1-B Babar Road, Block-B, Shaymali
Mohammadpur, Dhaka-1207
Bangladesh
Mobile: +08801912003485
Email: jaypeedhaka@gmail.com

Jaypee Brothers Medical Publishers (P) Ltd
Bhotahity, Kathmandu, Nepal
Phone: +977-9741283608
Email: kathmandu@jaypeebrothers.com

Website: www.jaypeebrothers.com
Website: www.jaypeedigital.com

© 2017, Jaypee Brothers Medical Publishers

The views and opinions expressed in this book are solely those of the original contributor(s)/author(s) and do not necessarily represent those of editor(s) of the book.

All rights reserved. No part of this publication may be reproduced, stored or transmitted in any form or by any means, electronic, mechanical, photocopying, recording or otherwise, without the prior permission in writing of the publishers.

All brand names and product names used in this book are trade names, service marks, trademarks or registered trademarks of their respective owners. The publisher is not associated with any product or vendor mentioned in this book.

Medical knowledge and practice change constantly. This book is designed to provide accurate, authoritative information about the subject matter in question. However, readers are advised to check the most current information available on procedures included and check information from the manufacturer of each product to be administered, to verify the recommended dose, formula, method and duration of administration, adverse effects and contraindications. It is the responsibility of the practitioner to take all appropriate safety precautions. Neither the publisher nor the author(s)/editor(s) assume any liability for any injury and/or damage to persons or property arising from or related to use of material in this book.

This book is sold on the understanding that the publisher is not engaged in providing professional medical services. If such advice or services are required, the services of a competent medical professional should be sought.

Every effort has been made where necessary to contact holders of copyright to obtain permission to reproduce copyright material. If any have been inadvertently overlooked, the publisher will be pleased to make the necessary arrangements at the first opportunity.

Inquiries for bulk sales may be solicited at: jaypee@jaypeebrothers.com

Clinic Consult Pulmonology: Tuberculosis

First Edition: **2017**

ISBN: 978-93-86322-01-2

Printed at: Samrat Offset Pvt. Ltd.

Preface

This handbook will be helpful to the practicing physicians dealing with management of tuberculosis. An attempt has been made to give precise information on the history, epidemiology, etiology, pathophysiology, clinical manifestations, and diagnosis of tuberculosis. Pertinent information on management issues are given that will help the physicians to make a quick decision for a proper prescription. Drug resistance and extrapulmonary tuberculosis are not discussed in detail as they will be taken up in subsequent and separate publications. Various illustrations and pictures incorporated in the book are from my personal collection and some are provided by Dr Amanjit Bal and Dr Mandeep Garg of my Institute. I am thankful to the Central Tuberculosis Division for allowing me to use and reproduce some of their data and recommendations in the Chapter on Revised National Tuberculosis Control Program. Last, but not the least, I express my sincere thanks to Jaypee Brothers Medical Publishers (P) Ltd. for taking up the task of publishing this book.

Digambar Behera

Contents

CHAPTER 1
History of Tuberculosis — 1

CHAPTER 2
Epidemiology — 9

CHAPTER 3
The Organism — 46

CHAPTER 4
Pathogenesis of Tuberculosis — 59

CHAPTER 5
Pathology of Tuberculosis — 82

CHAPTER 6
Clinical Presentation of Tuberculosis — 94

CHAPTER 7
Radiology of Tuberculosis — 107

CHAPTER 8
Laboratory Diagnosis of Tuberculosis — 122

CHAPTER 9
Antituberculosis Drugs 150

CHAPTER 10
Revised National Tuberculosis
Control Program of India 183

PLATE 1

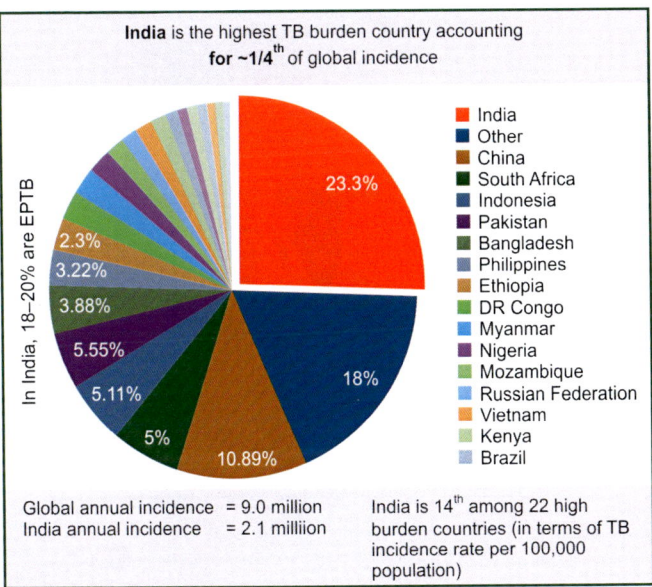

TB, tuberculosis, EPTB, extrapulmonary tuberculosis.

Figure 2.1 Tuberculosis incidence cases in 2013 in the 22 high burden countries. *(Chapter 2)*

Source: Global Tuberculosis Report 2014, World Health Organization.

PLATE 2

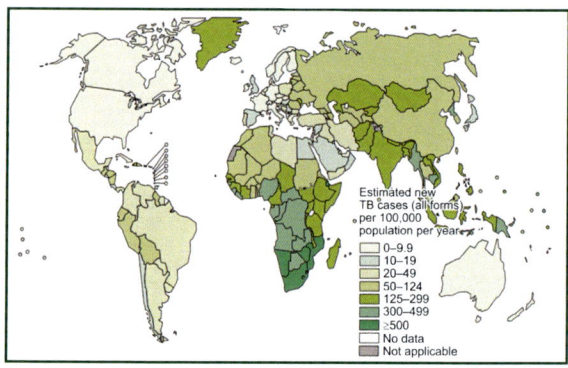

TB, tuberculosis.

Figure 2.3 Estimated tuberculosis incidence rates in 2013. *(Chapter 2)*
Source: Global Tuberculosis Report, 2014, World Health Organization.

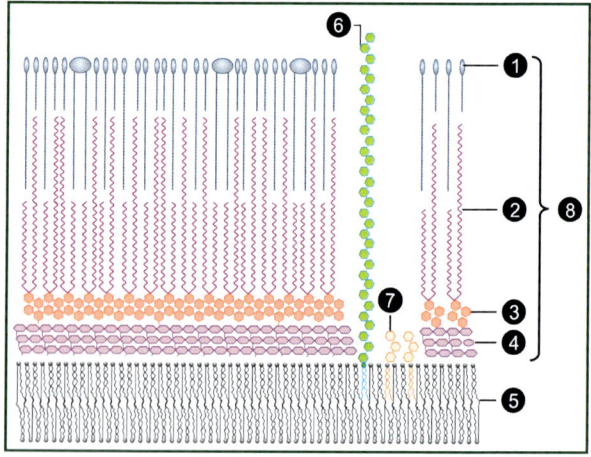

Figure 3.2 Mycobacterial cell wall. **1,** outer lipids; **2,** mycolic acid; **3,** polysaccharides (arabinogalactan); **4,** peptidoglycan; **5,** plasma membrane; **6,** lipoarabinomannan; **7,** phosphatidylinositol mannoside; **8,** cell wall skeleton. *(Chapter 3)*

PLATE 3

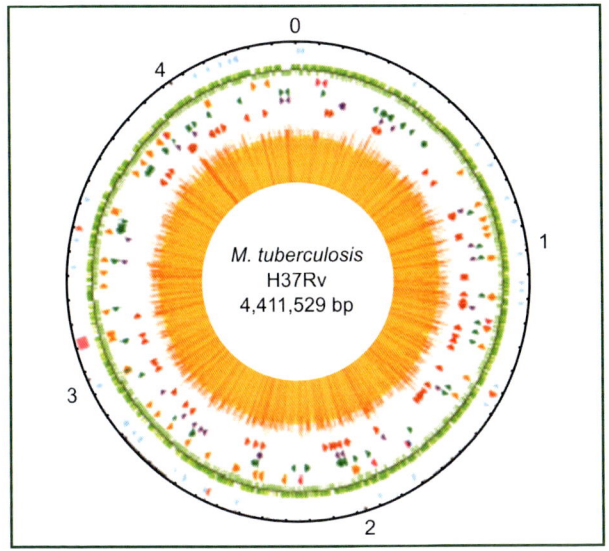

Figure 3.3 Circular map of the chromosome of *M. tuberculosis* H37Rv.*(Chapter 3)*

PLATE 4

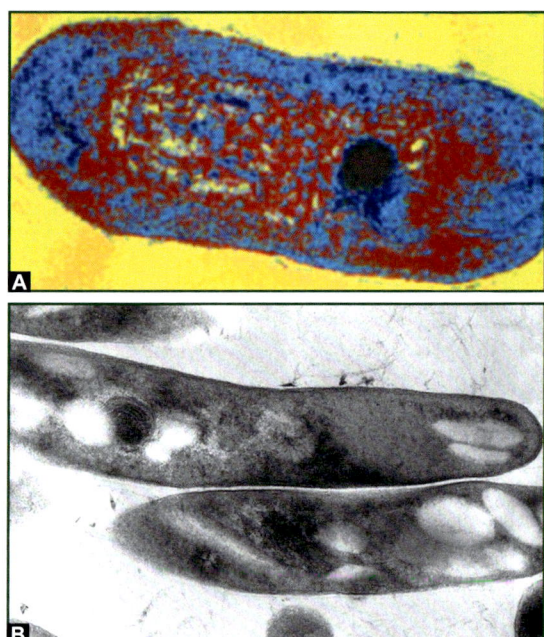

Figure 3.4 Electron micrograph of *Mycobacterium tuberculosis*. *(Chapter 3)*

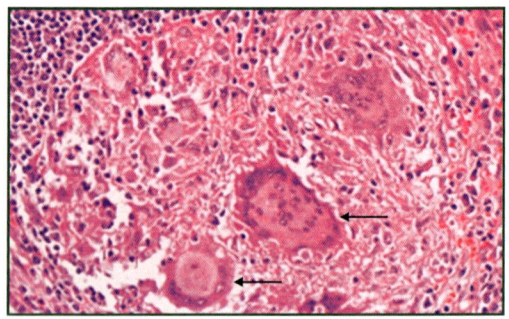

Figure 5.2 Granuloma and Langhan's giant cells. *(Chapter 5)*

PLATE 5

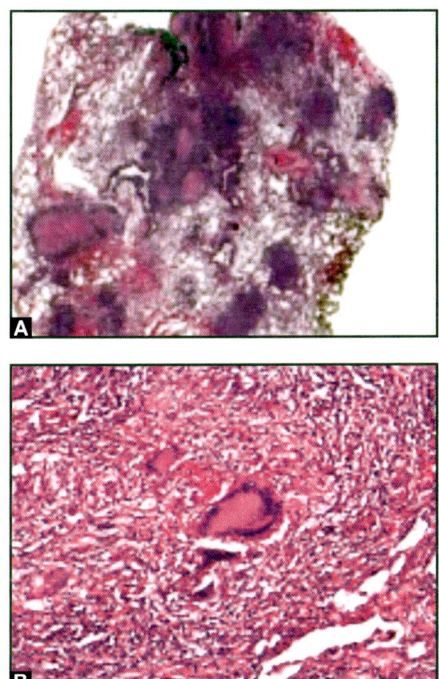

Figure 5.3 Tuberculous granuloma. *(Chapter 5)*

PLATE 6

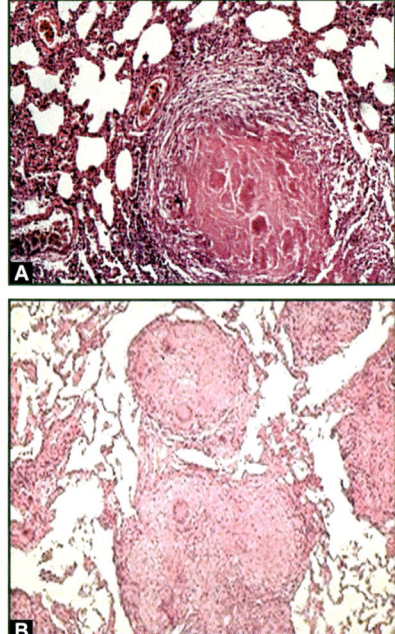

Figure 5.4 Granuloma of tuberculosis and sarcoidosis. *(Chapter 5)*

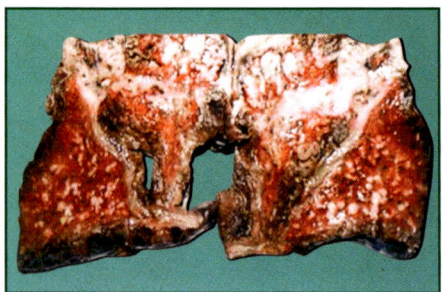

Figure 5.5 Fibrocaseous tuberculosis with cavitation (post-primary tuberculosis). *(Chapter 5)*

PLATE 7

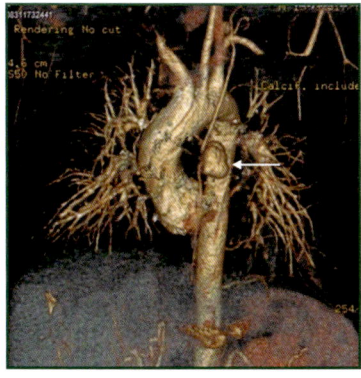

Figure 7.16 Reconstructed volume rendered image of computed tomography angiography showing pseudoaneurysm (arrow) arising from left internal mammary artery (LIMA) which was formed due to pocket of tubercular empyema located encasing the LIMA in the anterior aspect. *(Chapter 7)*

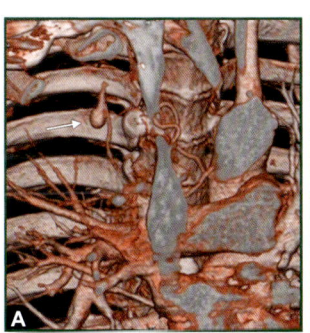
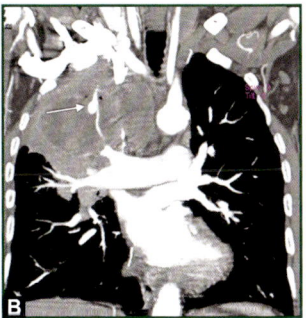
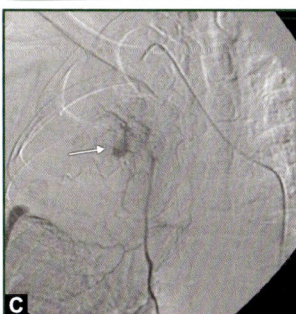

Figure 7.21 A, Volume rendering and **B,** coronal maximum intensity projection images showing a pseudoaneurysm in right upper lobe (arrows in A and B) arising from internal mammary artery (IMA). Surrounding consolidation is also seen. **C,** Selective right IMA run showing the pseudoaneurysm (arrow). *(Chapter 7)*

PLATE 8

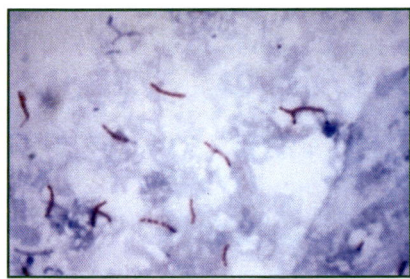

Figure 8.1 Acid-fast bacilli. Note red colored straight or slightly curved acid-fast bacilli. *(Chapter 8)*

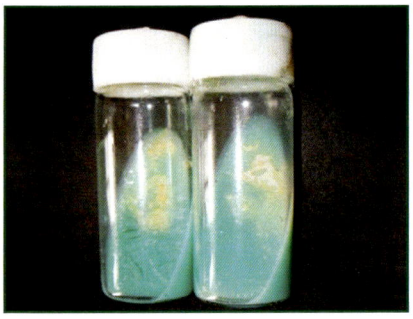

Figure 8.3 Note the growth of *Mycobacterium tuberculosis* in a Lowenstein Jensen media. *(Chapter 8)*

PLATE 9

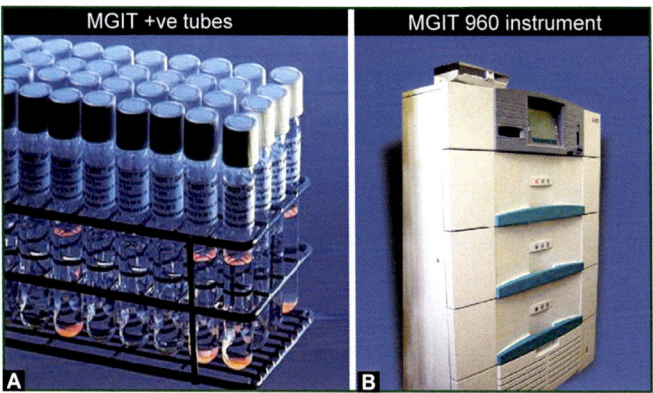

MGIT, mycobacteria growth indicator tube.

Figure 8.4 Mycobacterial growth indicator tube. *(Chapter 8)*

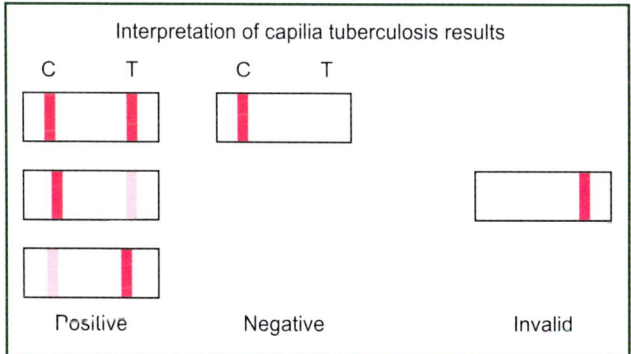

Figure 8.5 Capilia tuberculosis test to differentiate between species. *(Chapter 8)*

PLATE 10

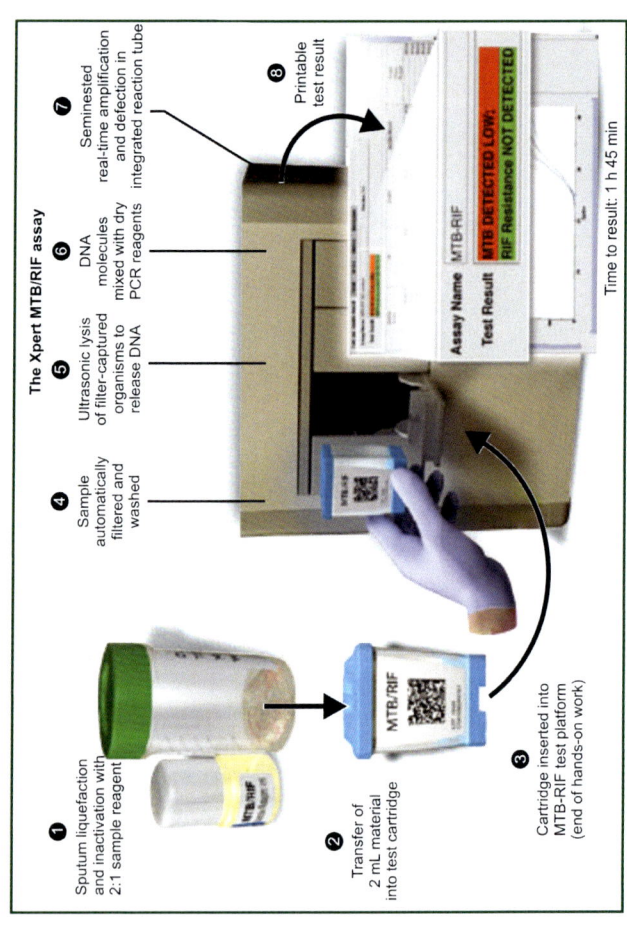

Figure 8.6 Gene'Xpert testing. (*Chapter 8*)

PLATE 11

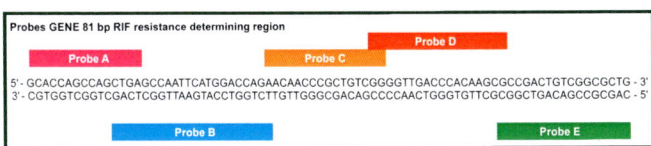

Figure 8.7: Gene probe for rifampicin resistance. *(Chapter 8)*

CHAPTER 1

History of Tuberculosis

Tuberculosis (TB) is a disease of antiquity that has long been a major public health challenge in the world, particularly in the developing countries. Early descriptions of the disease date to the pre-Christian era. Consumption, phthisis, scrofula, Pott's disease, and white plague are all terms used to refer to TB throughout history. It is postulated that humans first acquired the disease in Africa about 5,000 years ago. It spreads to other humans along trade routes. It also spread to domesticated animals, such as goats and cows, in Africa. Seals and sea lions that bred on African beaches are believed to have acquired the disease and carried it across the Atlantic to South America. Hunters would have been the first humans to contract the disease there.

The term "phthisis" first appeared in Greek literature around 460 BC. Hippocrates identified the illness as the most common cause of illness in his time. Although Aristotle believed that the disease might be contagious, many of his contemporaries believed it to be hereditary. Galen, the most eminent Greek physician after Hippocrates, defined phthisis as the ulceration of the lungs, thorax, or throat, accompanied by a cough, fever, and consumption of the body by pus. The TB epidemic in Europe, probably started in the 17th century, lasted 200 years, and was known as the "Great White Plague". Its incidence is thought to have peaked between the ends of 18th and 19th centuries. Over time, various cultures of the world gave the illness different names: *phthisis* (Greek), *consumption* (Latin), *yaksma* (India), and *chaky oncay* (Incan), each of which make reference to the "drying" or "consuming" aspects of the illness, cachexia. In the 19th century, TB's high mortality was referred to as the "romantic disease". The oldest example of spinal TB in the form of fossil bones dates back to about 8000 BC. Its evidenced in the mummified remains unearthed in Mesopotamia, Egypt and Central Asia, various Neolithic sites in Italy, Denmark, and countries in the Middle East. Europe become the epicenter for many TB epidemics starting in the 16th and 17th centuries due to population explosion and urbanization. European immigrants to the New World brought the disease with them.

Tuberculosis morbidity and mortality rates steadily dropped during the 20th century in the developed world as a result of better public health practices and widespread use of Bacillus Calmette-Guérin (BCG) vaccine, as well as the development of drugs in the 1950s. This downward trend ended and the numbers of new cases started increasing in the mid-1980s because of increased homelessness and poverty, and the emergence of human immunodeficiency virus (HIV)/acquired immune deficiency syndrome (HIV).

In 1865, Villemin, a French military physician, transmitted TB to laboratory rabbits by inoculating them with tuberculous tissue from a cadaver. He also demonstrated that environmental conditions greatly influenced the course of the disease. Dubos clearly rearticulated the role of environment. No specific class or strata in the society was immune to the disease. Death rate in the UK was 1% of the population by the 18th century due to TB and was known as "Captain of all these men of death" and "White Plague". Subsequently, the disease rose steadily for more than two centuries, but then it inexplicably went into a long, slow decline. Subsequent epidemiology of the disease varies according to the country, in some the decline was maintained, while in some others the rise continued with a plateau and then a decline till about a decade ago when it showed another rising trend because of the HIV infection. Royal touch was a form of treatment practiced in early days. Scrofula was known as the "mal du roi" or the "King's Evil". René Laennec, died from the disease at the age of 45, after contracting TB while studying contagious patients and infected bodies. He invented the stethoscope and used to corroborate his auscultatory findings. Another French physician Louis used statistical methods to evaluate different aspects of the disease's progression, the efficacy of various therapies, and individuals' susceptibility. He divided pthisis into six types. Koch, brought out major changes by establishing the basic and fundamental cause of TB in 1882. He delivered a lecture at the Physiological Society at the Christie Hospital, Berlin, on the 24th of March 1882 under the title *"Die Atiologie Tuberkulose"* and named the causative organism as the tubercle bacillus, the *Mycobacterium tuberculosis*. X-rays was discovered by von Rontgen in 1895. Scientific research of TB in the 19th century was more concerned with the description, pathogenesis, and diagnosis of the disease. The concept of sanatorium treatment started around the middle of 19th century. In the 1930s, collapse therapy through artificial pneumothorax and thoracoplasty supplemented due to discouraging results of sanatorium treatment.

Calmette and Guérin in 1906 developed the "BCG" vaccine from attenuated bovine-strain. The vaccine was first used on humans in 1921 in France, however, it was not until after World War II that BCG received widespread acceptance in the United States, Great Britain, and Germany. Bacillus Calmette-Guérin immunization was first carried out in Paris in 1921, which suffered a major setback in 1930 when

240 children were inadvertently vaccinated with virulent bacilli and 73 of them died. By 1945, BCG vaccination was again in use after its usefulness was realized. Modern drug treatment started with discovery of streptomycin in 1943 from the actinomycete, *Streptomyces griseus*. It was used for the first time on 20th November 1944 in a young woman. More discovery of many more anti-TB drugs was made: para-aminosalicylate sodium (PAS; 1949), isoniazid (1952), pyrazinamide (1954), cycloserine (1955), ethambutol (1962), rifampicin (1963), and more recently bedaquiline and others. From the use of monotherapy, the concept of combination therapy evolved, followed by domiciliary treatment and short-course chemotherapy.

The Modern Era

The modern era of TB control started in the mid-1990s when the World Health Organization (WHO) and various countries in the world adopted the directly observed treatment, short-course (DOTS) strategy. World Health Organization declared TB, a global public health emergency in 1993 and publishes a global report on TB every year since 1997. Stop TB Strategy, was launched in 2006 as an enhancement of the DOTS therapy.

HISTORY OF TUBERCULOSIS IN INDIA

The first references to TB in non-European civilization is found in the Vedas. The oldest of them (Rigveda, 1500 BC) calls the disease *yaksma*. The Atharvaveda calls it *balasa*. Atharvaveda gave the first description of scrofula. The *Sushruta Samhita* (600 BC) recommends treatment with breast milk, various meats, alcohol, and rest. The Yajurveda advises sufferers to move to higher altitudes.

Tuberculosis Control in India

The first open air sanatorium was founded in 1906 in Tiluania, near Ajmer, followed by one in Almora. In 1909, the first nonmissionary sanatorium was built near Shimla. United Mission Tuberculosis Sanatorium was built in 1912 at Madanapalle. Frimodt Moller, the first medical superintendent, played a large role in India's fight against TB through the training of TB workers, conducting TB surveys (1939), and introduction of BCG vaccination (1948). The first TB dispensary was opened in Bombay in 1917, followed by Madras. Soon anti-TB societies were formed in Lucknow and Ajmer. Government worked closely with the nongovernmental organizations and support their activities. The Tuberculosis Association of India (TAI) was formed in February, 1939. The provinces and states which received money also started their TB associations. The Bengal Tuberculosis Association had been functioning from 1929. In 1946, there were only 6,000 beds available for the treatment of TB patients. The Bhore Committee recommended enhancement. As no drug or combination of drugs were effective against TB till the middle of 20th century, the main line of treatment was good food, open air, and dry climate. Till the advent of adequate chemotherapy, treatment took a second place to diagnosis and prognosis. In 1939, the TAI recommended the Organized Home Treatment Scheme as the best compromise under the prevailing circumstances. Bacillus Calmette-Guérin work started in 1948; and in 1949, it was extended to schools in almost all the states of India. Under the aegis of the International Tuberculosis Campaign, which had considerable experience in BCG work in many countries, it was introduced in India on a small scale in Madanapalle with Frimodt Moller in the lead. India started a mass BCG campaign in 1951.

A BCG vaccine production center in Guindy, Madras, was set up in 1948 with WHO and United Nations Children's Fund support. In 1953, Frimodt Moller reported remarkable results with the regimen streptomycin (SM) and isoniazid (INH), single and combined, in the treatment of pulmonary TB in Indian patients. In 1956, Sikand and Pamra presented a paper on the "effect of SM, PAS, and INH in 703 cases of pulmonary TB, diagnosed and treated during 1951–53" and found that domiciliary treatment results were encouraging. The government established a Tuberculosis Chemotherapy Center in 1956 (Tuberculosis Research Center, in Madras, Chennai, now renamed as the National Institute of Research in Tuberculosis). It demonstrated that the time-honored virtues of sanatorium treatment such as bed rest, well-balanced diet, and good accommodation were remarkably unimportant provided adequate chemotherapy was prescribed and taken. Further, there was no evidence that close family contacts of patients treated at home incurred an increased risk of contracting TB. Therefore, it would be appropriate to treat infectious patients in their own homes. This finding revolutionized TB treatment the world over. National Tuberculosis Institute at Bangalore was established in 1959 for program and training. Countrywide national sample survey was carried out between 1955 and 1958 by the Indian Council of Medical Research. After a period of twelve and half years, it was shown that BCG vaccination did not offer significant protection against TB of the lung, but could provide substantial protection against childhood forms of TB such as tubercular meningitis and miliary TB. Bacillus Calmette-Guérin vaccination policy was revised and it was recommended to be given at an early age, preferably before the end of the first year after birth by integrating under Universal Immunization Program.

Evaluation of the National Tuberculosis Control Program

In 1992, the Government of India, together with the WHO and Swedish International Development Agency, reviewed the then national TB program and concluded that it suffered from managerial weakness, inadequate funding, over-reliance on X-ray, nonstandard treatment regimens, low rates of treatment completion, and lack of systematic information on treatment outcomes. As a result, a revised national tuberculosis control program was designed.

KEY MESSAGE

❑ Tuberculosis is a disease of antiquity that is known to exist for many centuries. It has devastated civilizations. The treatment and prevention attempts have failed earlier. Newer strategies in the form of TB control Programs are the new attempts to curtail the disease.

SUGGESTED READINGS

1. Andersen P. TB vaccines: progress and problems. Trends Immunol. 2002;22:160-8.
2. Barnes DS. Historical perspectives on the etiology of tuberculosis. Microbes Infect. 2000;2:431-40.
3. Dubos R, Dubos J. The White Plague: Tuberculosis, Man, and Society. Little Brown and Co.: Boston, MA; 1952.
4. Haas F, Hass SS. The origin of Mycobacterium tuberculosis and the notion of its contagiousness. In: Rom WN, Garay SM, editors. Tuberculosis. Little Brown and Co.: Boston, MA; 1996. pp. 3-19.
5. Herzog H. History of tuberculosis. Respiration. 1998;65:5-15.
6. Koch, R. 1882. Die Aetiologie der Tuberkulose. Berl. Klin. Wochenschr. 19:221-230. [Reprint, Am Rev Tuberc. 1932;25:285-323).

7. Morse D, Brothwell DR, Ucko PJ. Tuberculosis in ancient Egypt. Am Rev Respir Dis. 1964;90:524-41.
8. Reichman LB. The U-shaped curve of concern. Am Rev Respir Dis. 1991;144:741-2.
9. Ryan F. The forgotten plague. Little, Brown and Co.: Boston, MA; 1992.
10. Trudeau EL. Environment in its relation to the progress of bacterial invasion in tuberculosis. Am J Sci. 1887;94:118-23.

CHAPTER 2

Epidemiology

INTRODUCTION

The word epidemiology comes from the Greek words *epi*, meaning "on or upon", *demos*, meaning "people", and *logos*, meaning "the study of". It is the study of how often diseases occur in different groups of people and why. It also investigates all the factors that determine the presence or absence of diseases and disorders. About one-third of the global population (nearly 2 billion) is infected with tuberculosis (TB) and 95% of deaths due to TB are in the developing world. It is the second leading cause of death from an infectious disease worldwide after human immunodeficiency virus (HIV). Tuberculosis caused an estimated 1.5 million deaths in 2013 out of an estimated 9.0 million people who developed TB. Of these deaths, 360,000 were HIV-positive.

GLOBAL SCENE

Tuberculosis has been classically associated with poverty, overcrowding, and malnutrition. Mostly the young adults in their productive years are affected. Low income countries and deprived areas (particularly slums), within big cities in developed countries, present the highest TB incidences and TB mortality rates. These are settings where immigration, important social inequalities, HIV infection, and drug or alcohol abuse may coexist, all factors strongly associated with TB.

Epidemiology of TB will vary from country to country and from region to region. The epidemiology will also change from time to time depending on the time points of the study (like yearly and so on) because of varying control measures. Many earlier studies from different parts of the world have given varying figures. World Health Organization publishes a global TB report every year since 1997 to provide a comprehensive and up-to-date information of the TB epidemic situation and progress made in prevention, diagnosis, and treatment of the disease at global, regional, and country levels based primarily on data reported by countries and territories.

The 2014 global TB report is the 19th in the series of annual reports, and has used data from 202 countries and territories, including 183 member states, accounting for over 99% of the estimated world values. There are also other sources of estimation of the burden of disease.

The burden of disease caused by TB is expressed by three parameters:
1. Incidence: number of new and relapse cases arising in a given time period, usually 1 year
2. Prevalence: number of cases at a given point in time
3. Mortality: number of deaths caused by TB in a given time period, usually 1 year.

INCIDENCE

The 19th report of 2014 published in 2015, reported that, in 2013, there were an estimated 9.0 million (range, 8.6–9.4 million) incident cases (new and relapse cases) of TB,

Epidemiology

equivalent to 126 cases per 100,000 population. The absolute number of incident cases is falling slowly at an average rate of 1.5% per year between 2000 and 2013 and 0.6% between 2012 and 2013. The incidence in the 22 high burden countries is shown in Table 2.1 and depicted in Figure 2.1. Table 2.2 shows the burden in the six WHO regions of the world.

More than half of the estimated number of cases in 2013 reported are from Asia (South East and Western Pacific regions; 56%) and the African Region (29%).

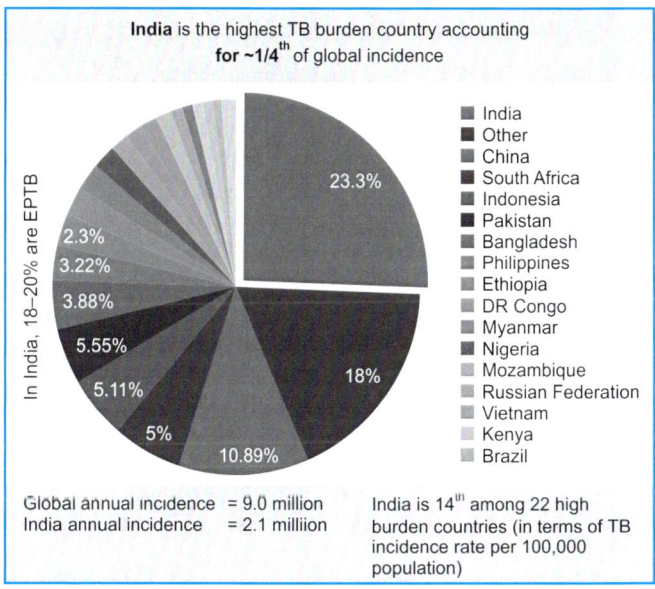

TB, tuberculosis, EPTB, extrapulmonary tuberculosis.

Figure 2.1 Tuberculosis incidence cases in 2013 in the 22 high burden countries. *(For color version, see Plate 1)*

Source: Global Tuberculosis Report 2014, World Health Organization.

TABLE 2.1

Estimated burden of tuberculosis (incidence, prevalence, and mortality) in 2013 in 22 high burden countries. Best estimates and lower and upper ranges of the 95% uncertainty interval (numbers in thousands[a])

Countries	Population	Prevalence		Incidence		Global burden (%)	HIV-positive incident TB cases		Mortality[b]		HIV-positive TB mortality	
India[c]	1,252,140	2,600	1,800–3,700	2,100	2,000–2,300	23.3	120	100–140	240	150–350	38	31–44
China	1,385,567	1,300	100–1,500	980	910–1,100	10.89	4.5	4.3–9.9	41	40–43	0.7	0.2–1.3
Nigeria	173,615	570	430–730	590	340–880	6.55	140	81–220	160	68–270	85	47–140
Pakistan	182,143	620	520–740	500	370–650	5.55	2.6	1.2–3.4	100	45–170	1	0.5–1.6
Indonesia[d]	249,866	680	340–1,100	460	410–520	5.11	15	8.7–20	64	36–93	3.9	2.2–6.2
South Africa	52,776	380	210–590	450	410–520	5.0	270	240–310	25	15–38	64	47–83
Bangladesh[e]	156,595	630	330–1,000	350	310–400	3.88	0.4	0.2–0.5	80	51–110	0.2	0.1–0.2
Philippines	98,394	430	380–490	290	260–330	3.22	0.3	0.2–0.3	27	25–29	<0.1	<0.1–<0.1
DR Congo	67,514	370	190–610	220	200–240	2.44	16	9.8–75	46	22–53	6.4	0.2–24

Continued

Continued

Estimated burden of tuberculosis (incidence, prevalence, and mortality) in 2013 in 22 high burden countries. Best estimates and lower and upper ranges of the 95% uncertainty interval (numbers in thousands[a])

Countries	Population	Prevalence		Incidence		Global burden (%)	HIV-positive incident TB cases	Mortality[b]		HIV-positive TB mortality	
Ethiopia	94,101	200	160–240	210	180–260	2.33	22	30	16–47	5.6	3.6–8.0
Myanmar	53,259	250	190–320	200	180–220	2.22	17	26	16–38	4.3	3.3–5.3
Mozambique	25,834	140	78–230	140	110–180	1.55	81	18	9.4–26	38	27–51
Russian Federation	142,834	160	74–290	130	120–140	1.44	7.9	17	17–18	1.4	1.0–1.9
Vietnam	91,680	190	79–350	130	110–160	1.44	9.4	17	12–24	2.0	1.2–2.9
Kenya	44,354	130	69–200	120	120–120	1.22	48	9.1	5.5–12	9.5	7.5–12
Brazil	200,362	110	54–200	93	83–110	1.03	13	4.4	2.5–6.8	2.1	1.5–2.7
UR Tanzania	49,253	85	45–140	81	77–84	0.90	30	6.0	3.4–8.2	6.1	4.8–7.5
Thailand	67,011	100	48–170	80	71–90	0.89	12	8.1	4.9–12	1.9	1.3–2.4
Zimbabwe	14,150	58	33–89	78	67–91	0.87	56	5.7	3.6–7.4	22	17–27
Uganda	37,579	58	32–91	62	56–73	0.68	32	4.1	2.2–6.6	7.2	5.0–9.9
Cambodia	15,135	110	91–130	61	55–67	0.68	2.3	10	6.3–14	0.6	0.5–0.8

Continued

Continued

Estimated burden of tuberculosis (incidence, prevalence, and mortality) in 2013 in 22 high burden countries. Best estimates and lower and upper ranges of the 95% uncertainty interval (numbers in thousands[a])

Countries	Population	Prevalence		Incidence		Global burden (%)	HIV-positive incident TB cases		Mortality[b]		HIV-positive TB mortality	
Afghanistan	30,552	100	54–170	58	51–65	0.64	0.2	0.2–0.2	13	8.4–16	<0.1	<0.1–0.1
TOTAL	4,434,710	9,300	8,200–11,000	7,400	7,100–7,800	–	910	820–990	960	810–1,100	300	250–350

TB, tuberculosis; HIV, human immunodeficiency virus; ICD, International Classifications of Diseases.

a. Numbers for mortality, prevalence, and incidence shown to two significant figures. Totals (high burden countries, regional and global) are computed prior to rounding.

b. Mortality excludes deaths among HIV-positive TB cases. Deaths among HIV-positive TB cases are classified as HIV deaths according to ICD-10 and are shown separately in this table.

c. Estimates for India have not yet been officially approved by the Ministry of Health & Family Welfare, Government of India, and should therefore be considered provisional.

d. As this report went to press, estimates for Indonesia were being revised based on the results of the 2013–2014 national TB prevalence survey. Updated estimates will be published online.

e. Estimates of TB disease burden have not been approved by the national TB program in Bangladesh and a joint reassessment will be undertaken following completion of the prevalence survey planned for 2015.

TABLE 2.2

Burden of tuberculosis in 2013 in different World Health Organization (WHO) regions of the world (Global Tuberculosis Report, 2014, WHO)

WHO regions	Population	Prevalence		Incidence		Global burden (%)	HIV-positive incident TB cases		Mortality*		HIV-positive TB mortality	
SEAR	1,855,068	4,500	3,500–5,700	3,400	3,200–3,600	37.77	170	150–190	440	330–550	48	42–55
AFR	927,371	2,800	2,400–3,200	2,600	2,300–2,900	28.88	870	790–960	390	300–500	300	250–350
WPR	1,858,410	2,300	2,000–2,500	1,600	1,500–1,700	17.77	23	19–26	110	100–120	4.8	3.7–5.9
EMR	616,906	1,000	880–1,200	750	620–890	8.33	5.1	4.0–6.4	140	90–210	1.8	1.3–2.4
EUR	907,053	460	350–590	360	340–370	4.00	21	20–22	38	37–39	3.8	3.2–4.4
AMR	970,821	370	290–460	280	270–300	3.11	32	31–33	14	12–17	6.1	5.5–6.8
Global	7,135,628	11,000	10,000–13,000	9,000	8,600–9,400	–	1,100	1,000–1,200	1,100	980–1,300	360	310–410

WHO, World Health Organization; TB, tuberculosis; HIV, human immunodeficiency virus; SEAR, South East Asia region; AFR, Africa region, WPR, Western Pacific region; EMR, Eastern Mediterranean region; EUR, Europe region; AMR, Americas region.

*Mortality excludes deaths among HIV-positive TB cases. Deaths among HIV-positive TB cases are classified as HIV deaths according to ICD-10 and are shown separately in this table.

The six countries having the largest number of cases in 2013 were:
- India (2–2.3 million)
- China (0.9–1.1 million)
- Nigeria (340,000 – 880,000)
- Pakistan (370,000 – 650,000)
- Indonesia (410,000 – 520,000)
- South Africa (410,000 – 520,000).

These and the other five countries that make up the top ten in terms of numbers of cases are highlighted in Figure 2.2. India and China alone accounted for 24 and 11% of global cases, respectively. Of the 9.0 million incident cases, an estimated 550,000 were children and 3.3 million (range, 3.2–3.5 million) occurred among women. The 9.0 million incident TB cases in 2013 included 1.0 million–1.2 million (11–14%) among people living with HIV with a best estimate of 1.1 million (13%).

The estimated burden of TB per 100,000 population in the 22 high burden countries and six WHO regions is shown in Table 2.3.

The latest assessment for the 22 high burden countries suggests that incidence rates are falling in most countries (Figures 2.3–2.5).

PREVALENCE

There were an estimated 11 million prevalent cases (range, 10 million–13 million) of TB in 2013 in the world (Table 2.1), equivalent to 159 cases per 100,000 population (Table 2.2). By 2013, the prevalence rate had fallen 41% globally since 1990. Current forecasts suggest that the Stop TB Partnership target of halving TB prevalence by 2015 compared with a baseline of 1990 will not be met worldwide (Figure 2.5).

Regionally, prevalence rates are declining in all six WHO regions. The Americas region has halved the 1990 level of TB prevalence by around 2005, well in advance of the target year

Epidemiology

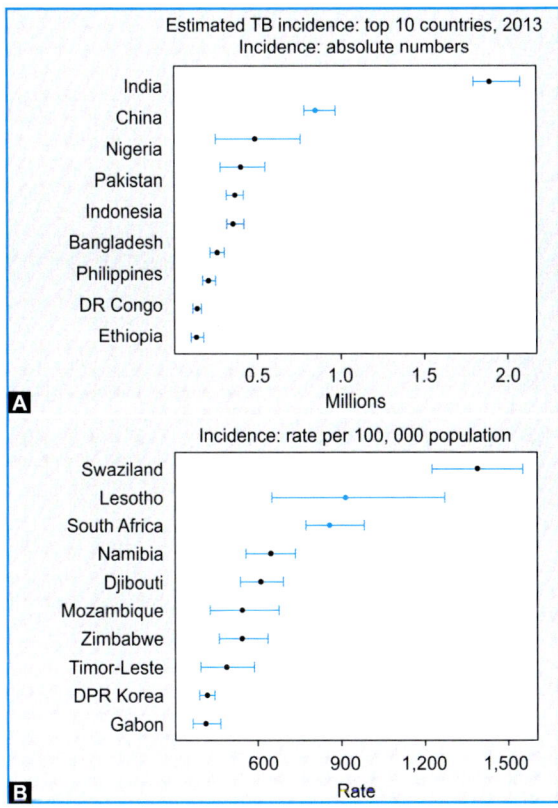

TB, tuberculosis.

Figure 2.2 Tuberculosis incidence in the **A,** highest 10 countries of the world and **B,** incidence rates per 100,000 population.

Source: Global Tuberculosis Report, 2014, World Health Organization.

of 2015, and the best estimate suggests that the Western Pacific Region would achieved the 50% reduction target in 2012. Reaching the 50% reduction target by 2015 appears feasible

TABLE 2.3

Estimated tuberculosis burden in 2013 per 100,000 population. Best estimates are followed by the lower and upper bounds of the 95% uncertainty interval (Global Tuberculosis Report, 2014, World Health Organization)

	Population (thousands)	Mortality[a]		HIV-positive TB mortality		Prevalence		Incidence		HIV prevalence in incident TB cases (%)	
Afghanistan	30,552	42	27–53	0.3	0.2–0.3	340	178–554	189	167–212	0.34	0.29–0.40
Bangladesh[b]	156,595	51	33–69	0.1	<0.1–0.2	402	210–656	224	199–253	0.12	<0.1–0.16
Brazil	200,362	2.2	1.3–3.4	1.0	0.8–1.4	57	27–99	46	41–52	14	13–16
Cambodia	15,135	66	42–92	3.9	3.0–5.0	715	604–834	400	366–444	3.9	3.4–4.4
China	1,385,567	3.0	2.9–3.1	<0.1	<0.1–0.1	94	82–107	70	66–77	0.46	0.22–0.79
DR Congo	67,514	68	33–78	9.5	0.3–35	549	285–898	326	297–356	7.5	0.13–27
Ethiopia	94,101	32	17–50	5.9	3.8–8.5	211	170–257	224	188–276	11	7.4–14
India[c]	1,252,140	19	12–28	3.0	2.5–3.5	211	143–294	171	162–184	5.7	4.8–6.6
Indonesia[d]	249,866	25	14–37	1.6	0.9–2.5	272	138–450	183	164–207	3.2	2.1–4.5
Kenya	44,354	20	12–27	21	17–27	283	156–447	268	261–275	41	39–42
Mozambique	25,834	69	36–101	148	105–198	559	303–893	552	442–680	57	39–74
Myanmar	53,259	49	29–71	8.0	6.3–9.9	473	364–595	373	340–413	8.8	7.8–9.8
Nigeria	173,615	94	39–156	49	27–78	326	246–418	338	194–506	25	10–44
Pakistan	182,143	56	25–92	0.5	0.3–0.9	342	284–406	275	205–357	0.53	0.3–0.83

Continued

Continued

Epidemiology

Estimated tuberculosis burden in 2013 per 100,000 population. Best estimates are followed by the lower and upper bounds of the 95% uncertainty interval (Global Tuberculosis Report, 2014, World Health Organization)

	Population (thousands)	Mortality[a]		HIV-positive TB mortality		Prevalence		Incidence		HIV prevalence in incident TB cases (%)	
Philippines	98,394	27	25–29	<0.1	<0.1–<0.1	438	385–495	292	261–331	0.11	<0.1–0.14
Russian Federation	142,834	12	12–13	1.0	0.7–1.3	114	51–201	89	82–100	6.2	5.2–7.3
South Africa	52,776	48	28–73	121	90–158	715	396–1130	860	776–980	61	50–71
Thailand	67,011	12	7.3–18	2.8	2.0–3.6	149	72–252	119	106–134	15	12–17
Uganda	37,579	11	5.8–18	19	13–26	154	85–243	166	149–193	52	42–62
UR Tanzania	49,253	12	7.0–17	12	9.8–15	172	92–277	164	157–170	37	35–39
Viet Nam	91,680	19	13–26	2.1	1.3–3.2	209	86–384	144	121–174	7.2	5.4–9.1
Zimbabwe	14,150	40	25–52	153	121–189	409	235–630	552	474–643	72	55–86
High-burden countries	**4,484,710**	**21**	**18–25**	**6.7**	**5.6–7.9**	**208**	**183–235**	**165**	**158–173**	**12**	**11–14**
AFR	927,371	42	32–54	32	27–38	300	263–341	280	251–311	34	29–39
AMR	970,821	1.5	1.2–1.7	0.6	0.6–0.7	38	30–48	29	28–31	11	11–12
EMR	616,906	23	15–34	0.3	0.2–0.4	165	143–189	121	100–144	0.94	0.67–1.2

Continued

Continued

Estimated tuberculosis burden in 2013 per 100,000 population. Best estimates are followed by the lower and upper bounds of the 95% uncertainty interval (Global Tuberculosis Report, 2014, World Health Organization)

	Population (thousands)	Mortality[a]		HIV-positive TB mortality		Prevalence		Incidence		HIV prevalence in incident TB cases (%)	
EUR	907,053	4.1	4.0–4.2	0.4	0.4–0.5	51	39–65	39	38–41	6.0	5.6–6.4
SEAR	1,855,068	23	18–30	2.6	2.2–3.0	244	188–307	183	175–192	4.9	4.4–5.5
WPR	1,858,410	5.8	5.4–6.3	0.3	0.2–0.3	121	109–134	87	82–92	1.4	1.2–1.6
Global	7,135,628	16	14–18	5.0	4.3–5.8	159	143–176	126	121–131	13	12–14

WHO, World Health Organization; TB, tuberculosis; HIV, human immunodeficiency virus; SEAR, South East Asia region; AFR, Africa region, WPR, Western Pacific region; EMR, Eastern Mediterranean region; EUR, Europe region; AMR, Americas region.

[a]Mortality excludes deaths among HIV-positive TB cases. Deaths among HIV-positive TB cases are classified as HIV deaths according to ICD-10 and are shown separately in this table.

[b]Estimates of TB disease burden have not been approved by the national TB program in Bangladesh and a joint reassessment will be undertaken following completion of the prevalence survey planned for 2015.

[c]Estimates for India have not yet been officially approved by the Ministry of Health and Family Welfare, Government of India, and should therefore be considered provisional.

[d]As this report went to press, estimates for Indonesia were being revised based on the results of the 2013–2014 national TB prevalence survey. Updated estimates will be published online by WHO in 2015.

Epidemiology

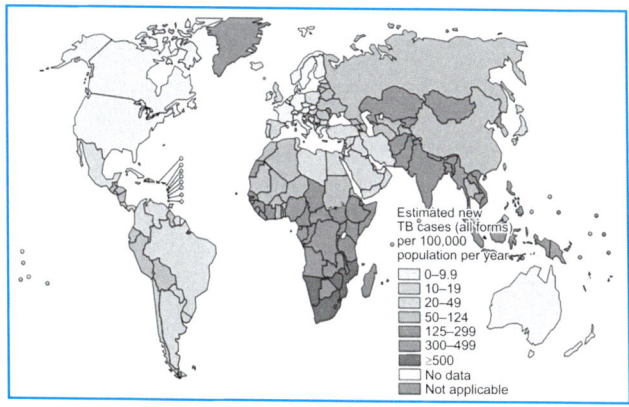

TB, tuberculosis.

Figure 2.3 Estimated tuberculosis incidence rates in 2013. *(For color version, see Plate 2)*
Source: Global Tuberculosis Report, 2014, World Health Organization.

in the South East Asia region as well. The target appears out of reach in the African, European, and Eastern Mediterranean regions (Figure 2.6).

MORTALITY

An estimated 1.5 million TB deaths occurred in 2013 (Table 2.1), of which 1.1 million was among HIV-negative people and 360,000 among HIV-positive people (Figure 2.7). These deaths included 510,000 among women and 80,000 among children. There were approximately 210,000 deaths from multidrug-resistant (MDR)-TB (range, 30,000–290,000). Approximately 78% of total TB deaths and 73% of TB deaths among HIV-negative people occurred in the African and South East Asia regions in 2013. India and Nigeria accounted for about one-third of global TB deaths. An average of 15 deaths per 100,000 population of the world was due to TB in 2013

Clinic Consult Pulmonology: Tuberculosis

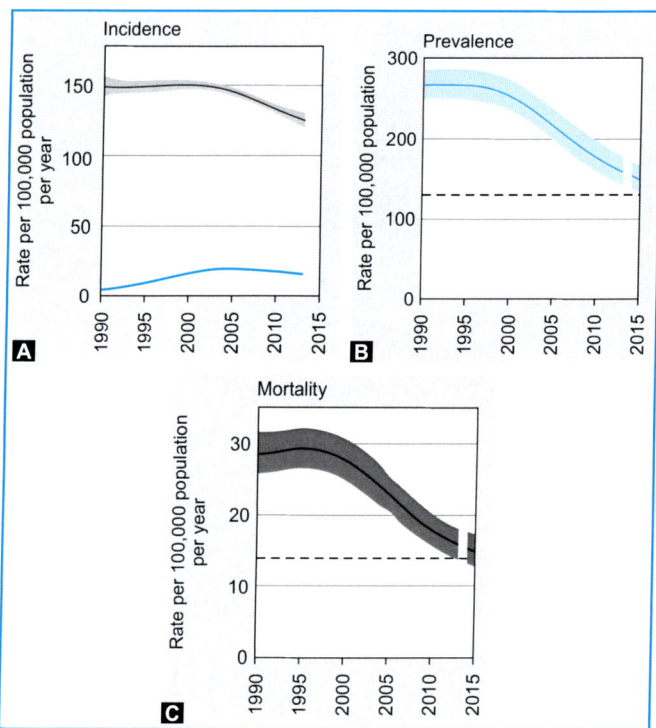

Figure 2.4 Global trends of estimated incidence rates, prevalence rates, and mortality rates. **A,** Global trends in estimated incidence rates including human immunodeficiency virus (HIV)-positive tuberculosis (TB) (in black) and estimated rates in HIV-positive TB (in blue). **B,** Trends in estimated prevalence rate between 1990 and 2013 and forecast rates between 2014 and 2015. **C,** Trends in estimated mortality rate between 1990 and 2013 and forecast rates between 2014 and 2015. The horizontal dashed lines represents the Stop TB Partnership targets of a 505 reduction in prevalence and mortality rates by 2015 compared to 1990. Shaded areas in all pictures represent uncertainty bands. Mortality excludes TB deaths among HIV-positive people.

Source: Global tuberculosis report, 2014, World Health Organization.

Epidemiology

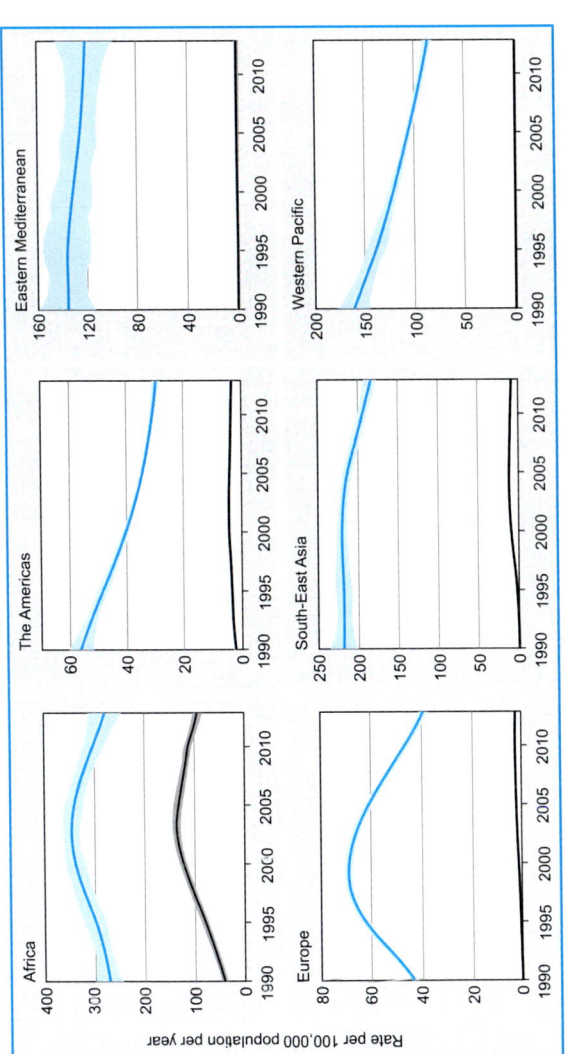

Figure 2.5 Tuberculosis incidence rates (per 100,000 population) in World Health Organization regions between 1990 and 2013. Regional trends are shown in blue and that in HIV-positive cases shown in black. Shaded areas represent uncertainty bands.

Source: Global Tuberculosis Report, 2014, World Health Organization.

Clinic Consult Pulmonology: Tuberculosis

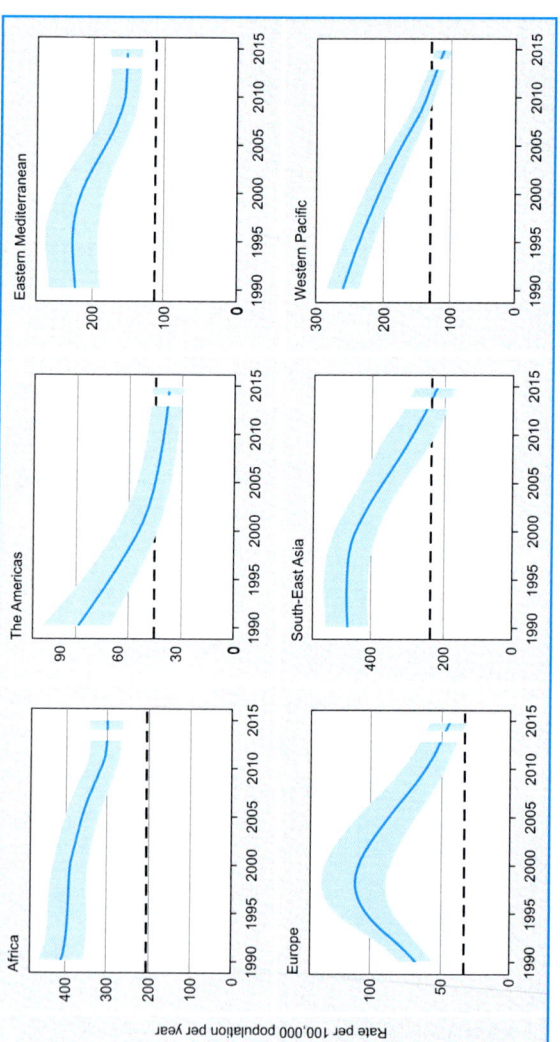

Figure 2.6 Trends in estimated tuberculosis prevalence rates 1990–2013 and forecast tuberculosis (TB) prevalence rates 2014–2015 by World Health Organization region. Shaded areas represent uncertainty bands. The horizontal dashed lines represent the Stop TB Partnership target of a 50% reduction in the prevalence rate by 2015 compared with 1990. The other dashed lines show projections up to 2015.

Source: Global Tuberculosis Report, 2014, World Health Organization.

Epidemiology

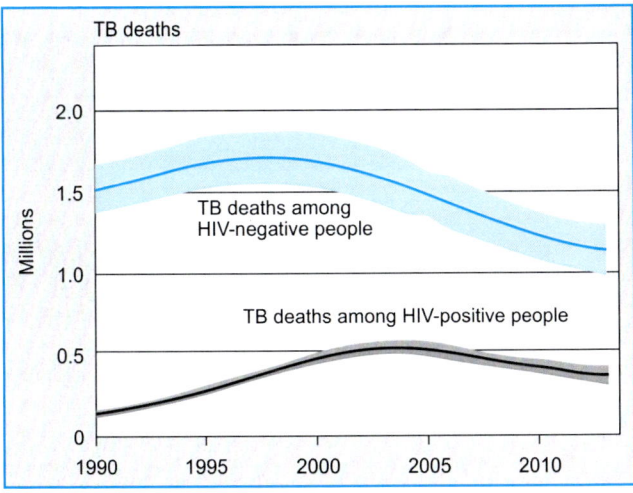

TB, tuberculosis; HIV, human immunodeficiency virus.

Figure 2.7 Absolute estimated tuberculosis deaths (in millions) between 1990 and 2013.

Source: Global Tuberculosis Report, 2014, World Health Organization.

(Table 2.2) and 21 when TB deaths among HIV-positive people are included. Globally, the mortality rate (excluding deaths among HIV-positive people) has fallen by 45% between 1990 and 2013.

The current rate of decline will need to accelerate to reach the Stop TB Partnership target of a 50% reduction by 2015 (Figure 2.5). Regionally, mortality rates are declining in all six WHO regions. The 2015 target has already been surpassed in the Americas (since 2004) and the Western Pacific (since 2002) regions, and may have been reached in 2013 in the South East Asia region. Between 2000 and 2013, TB diagnostic and treatment interventions saved an estimated 37 million lives (Tables 2.4 and 2.5).

TABLE 2.4

Cumulative lives saved by tuberculosis prevention, diagnosis, and treatment interventions between 2000 and 2013 in the world and the World Health Organization (WHO) regions in millions. Best estimates are followed by uncertainty intervals (Global Tuberculosis Report, 2014, WHO)

Region	HIV-negative		HIV-positive		Total	
AFR	4.0	3.3–4.8	5.0	4.5–5.6	9.1	8.1–10
AMR	1.4	1.2–1.5	0.28	0.26–0.30	1.6	1.5–1.8
EMR	2.6	2.1–3.0	0.03	0.026–0.034	2.6	2.2–3.1
EUR	2.1	1.8–2.3	0.15	0.14–0.16	2.2	2.0–2.4
SEAR	11	9.7–13	1.0	0.91–1.1	12	11–14
WPR	8.7	7.9–9.6	0.14	0.13–0.16	8.9	8.0–9.7
Global	30	26–34	7.0	6.3–7.7	37	33–41

HIV, human immunodeficiency virus; AFR, Africa region, AMR, Americas region; EMR, Eastern Mediterranean region; EUR, Europeregion; SEAR, South East Asia region; WPR, Western Pacific region.

TABLE 2.5

Case fatality ratios in the absence of treatment	
Tuberculosis cases	Case fatality ratio (range)
HIV-negative not on TB treatment	0.43 (0.28–0.53)
HIV-positive not on ART, not on TB treatment	0.78 (0.65–0.94)

HIV, human immunodeficiency virus; TB, tuberculosis; ART, Antiretroviral therapy.

TUBERCULOSIS IN WOMEN AND CHILDREN

There were an estimated 3.3 million new cases of TB and 510,000 deaths from the disease among women in 2013. Among children, there were an estimated 550,000 new cases in 2013 and 80,000 deaths among children who were HIV-negative. The African and South East Asia regions account for 69% of the cases among women. The incidence in women and children is shown in Table 2.6.

TABLE 2.6

Total number of new and relapsed cases of tuberculosis notifications and estimated incident cases among women in 2013 globally and for the World Health Organization (WHO) regions (Global Tuberculosis Report, 2014, WHO)

WHO region	Number of tuberculosis case notifications among women	Estimated tuberculosis incidence among women	
		Best estimate	Uncertainty interval
AFR	390,808	990,000	880,000–1,100,000
AMR	73,905	100,000	96,000–110,000
EMR	180,917	330,000	270,000–390,000
EUR	84,508	120,000	110,000–130,000
SEAR	234,190	1,300,000	1,200,000–1,400,000
WPR	346,537	510,000	480,000–530,000
Global	1,310,865	3,300,000	3,200,000–3,500,000

WHO, World Health Organization; AFR, Africa region, AMR, Americas region; EMR, Eastern Mediterranean region; EUR, Europe region; SEAR, South East Asia region; WPR, Western Pacific region.

MULTIDRUG-RESISTANT TUBERCULOSIS

About 480,000 people developed multidrug-resistant tuberculosis (MDR-TB) in the world in 2013. More than half of these cases were in India, China, and the Russian Federation. It is estimated that about 9.0% of MDR-TB cases had extensively drug-resistant (XDR)-TB.

In 2013, the average proportion of MDR-TB cases with XDR-TB was 9.0%. The proportion of MDR-TB cases with XDR-TB was highest in Georgia (20.0%), Kazakhstan (22.7%), Latvia (21.7%), Lithuania (24.8%), and Tajikistan (Dushanbe city and Rudaki district: 21.0%). By the end of June 2015, 104 countries had notified at least one case of XDR-TB. The MDR-/XDR-TB are discussed in more detail in part II of the series.

GLOBAL BURDEN OF DISEASE STUDY

While most of the information presented above is from the WHO data, the Global Burden of Disease study has presented a slightly different figures for incidence, prevalence of mortality from TB. The results are given in Table 2.7. The global TB situation in 2013 is summarized in Table 2.8.

TABLE 2.7

All forms of tuberculosis in both human immunodeficiency virus (HIV)-positive and HIV-negative cases (The Global Burden of Disease Study)	
Incidence	7.5 million (7.4 million to 7.7 million)
Prevalence	11.9 million (11.6 million to 12.2 million)
Death	1.4 million (1.3 million to 1.5 million)

TABLE 2.8

Global tuberculosis in 2013 (report on Global Burden of Tuberculosis, 2014, World Health Organization)		
	Estimated incidence, 2013	*Estimated number of deaths, 2013*
All forms of TB	9.0 million (8.6–9.4 million) (rate 126)	1.1 milion* (1.0–1.3 million)
HIV-associated TB	1.1 million (1.0–1.2 million)	360,000 (310,000–410,000)
Multidrug-resistant TB	480,000 (350,000–610,000) 300,000 (230,000–380,000) amongst notified cases	210,000 (130,000–290,000)

HIV, human immunodeficiency virus; TB, tuberculosis.
Source: World Health Organization Global Tuberculosis Report, 2014.

INDIAN SCENARIO

There was paucity of information on the true burden of TB disease in the country although considerable light was thrown on the epidemiology in India by studies reported in early 40s. The first ever National Sample Survey of TB conducted by Indian Council of Medical Research in 1955–58 revealed that the prevalence of sputum positive pulmonary TB is about 4 per 1,000 population and an estimated 1.5 million infectious cases spreading infection in the community.

Subsequently, many other surveys including the prevalence of infection, annual risk of TB infection (ARTI), and clinical, radiological, and bacteriological prevalence of TB were carried out. These were subsequently discarded, as there were many flaws in these estimates and they did not reflect a correct picture of the TB situation in the country. The incidence of TB in India is estimated based on findings of nationwide ARTI study conducted in 2000–03. The national ARTI being 1.5%, the incidence of new smear positive TB cases in the country is estimated as 75 new smear positive cases per 100,000 populations.

The Central TB Division of the Government of India prepares its annual report each year from many years now which gives an account of various aspects of TB in the country, including the reported cases, its own "Nikshay" project which is a case based online software and reported and recorded cases presented to the program (Figure 2.8).

The 2015 Annual Report as well as the Global report shows that:
- India is the highest TB burden country in the world having more new cases annually than any other country. Although it is the second-most populous country in the world, nearly one-fourth of the global incident TB cases occur in India annually (Figure 2.1). In 2013, out of the estimated global

Clinic Consult Pulmonology: Tuberculosis

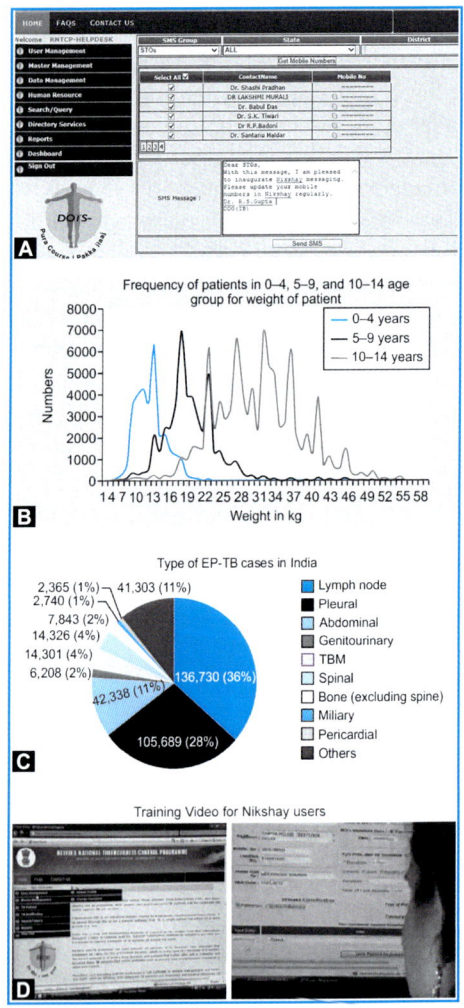

Figure 2.8 Nikshay: case-based-web-based recording and reporting system.

annual incidence of 9 million TB cases, 2.1 million were estimated to have occurred in India. The overall burden of TB (incidence, prevalence, and mortality), HIV-TB, and MDR-TB in 2013 in India is shown in Table 2.9

- There is 50% reduction in TB mortality rate by 2013 compared to 1990 level
- There is 55% reduction in TB prevalence rate by 2013 compared to 1990 level.

These estimations were based on Revised National Tuberculosis Control Program (RNTCP) data, seven prevalence surveys in India conducted between 2007 and 2010, national ARTI surveys, and mortality surveys conducted in 2005. Tuberculosis prevalence per lakh population has reduced from 465 in year 1990 to 211 in 2013. In absolute numbers,

TABLE 2.9

Tuberculosis (TB) burden in India in 2013 (Annual TB Report 2015, Central TB Division, Government of India)		
TB burden	Number (millions) (95% CI)	Rate per 100,000 persons (95% CI)
Incidence	2.1 (2.0–2.3)	171 (162–184)
Prevalence	2.6 (1.8–3.7)	211 (143–294)
Mortality	0.24 (0.15–0.35)	19 (12–28)
HIV among estimated incident TB patients		5.7% (4.8–6.6%)
MDR-TB among notified pulmonary TB patients	0.062 (0.050–0.074)	
MDR-TB among notified new pulmonary TB patients	0.020 (0.018–0.025)	2.2% (1.9–2.6%)
MDR-TB among notified retreatment pulmonary TB patients	0.042 (0.033–0.054)	15% (11–19%)

TB, tuberculosis; HIV, human immunodeficiency virus; MDR, mutidrug-resistant; CI, confidence interval.

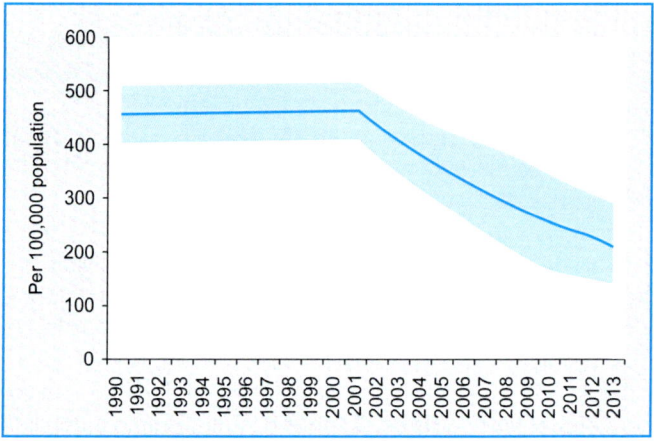

Figure 2.9 Prevalence of tuberculosis in India over the years (1990–2013).

prevalence has reduced from 40 lakhs to 26 lakhs annually (Figure 2.9).

Tuberculosis incidence per lakh population has reduced from 216 in year 1990 to 171 in 2013 (Figure 2.10).

Tuberculosis mortality per lakh population has reduced from 38 in year 1990 to 19 in 2012. In absolute numbers, morality due to TB has reduced from 3.3 lakhs to 2.4 lakhs annually (Figure 2.11).

As per the RNTCP data, the prevalence and mortality are reducing as per the Millennium Development Goal (MDG) guidelines and the program is doing well. Impact of RNTCP is shown in Figure 2.12.

Since the inception of RNTCP in 1997, the program has diagnosed and treated more than 17.4 million TB cases and 3.1 million additional lives have been saved. In line with the MDGs, TB prevalence has been reduced from 465/100,000

Epidemiology

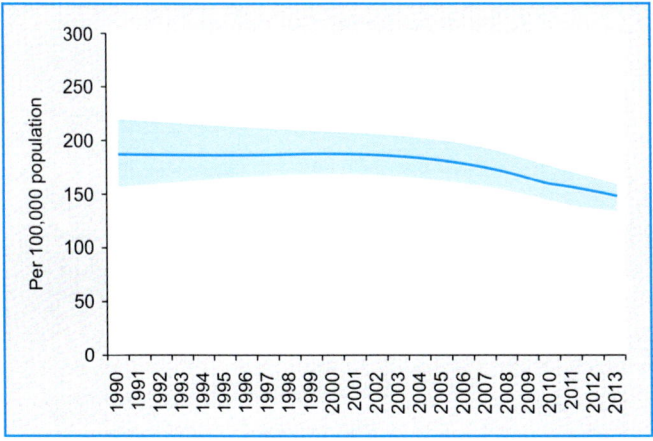

Figure 2.10 Incidence of tuberculosis in India over the years (1990–2013).

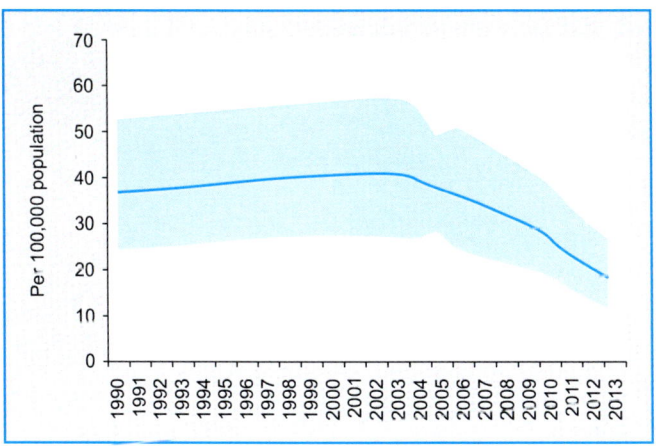

Figure 2.11 Mortality of tuberculosis in India over the years (1990–2013).

Clinic Consult Pulmonology: Tuberculosis

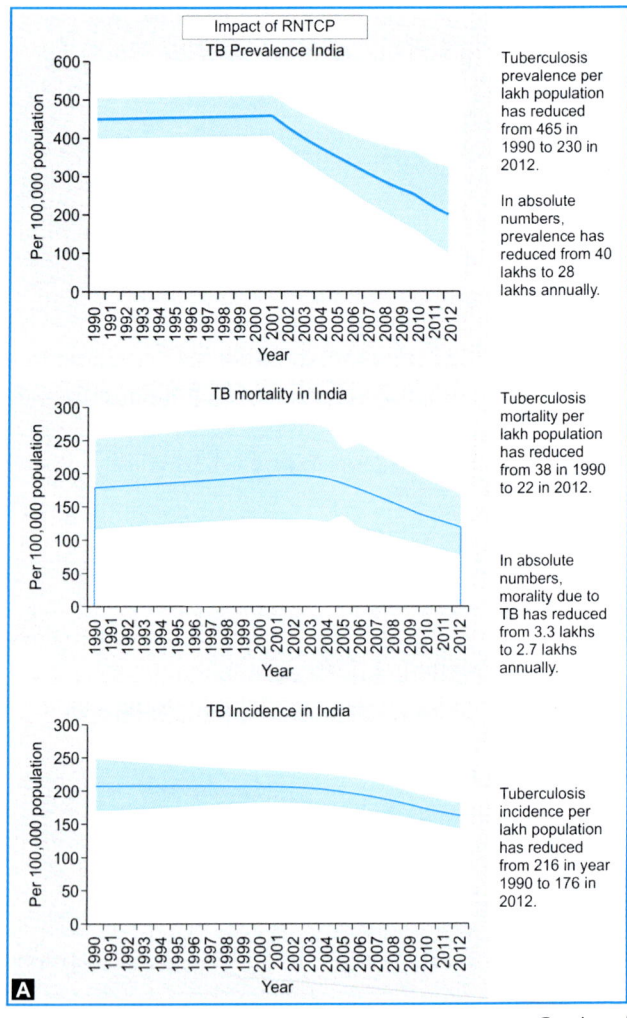

Continued

Continued

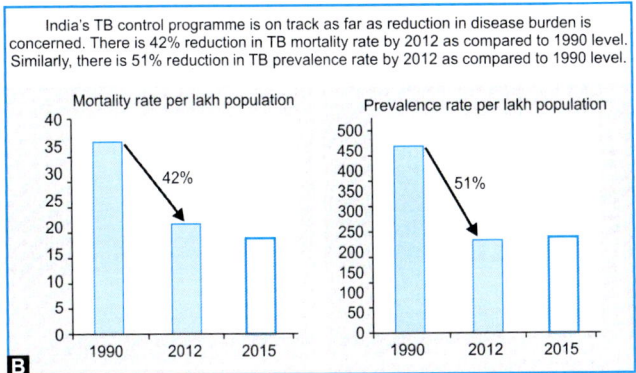

RNTCP, Revised National Tuberculosis Control Program; TB, tuberculosis.

Figure 2.12 Impact of Revised National Tuberculosis Control Program on tuberculosis epidemiology in India.

per year in 1990 to 211/100,000 per year in 2013. The incidence of TB has reduced from 216/100,000 per year in 1990 to 171/100,000 per year in 2013 and mortality from 38/100,000 per year in 1990 to 19/100,000 per year in 2013. The estimates of TB burden in 2013 in India is summarized in Table 2.10.

It is summarized in Tables 2.11 and 2.12.

TUBERCULOSIS-HUMAN IMMUNODEFICIENCY VIRUS IN INDIA

Prevalence of *Mycobacterium tuberculosis*/HIV coinfection worldwide was 0.18% and 640,000 incident TB cases (8%) had HIV infection in 2007. The case fatality rate was very high (exceeding >50%) in some African countries. The global estimation of burden of HIV-positive incident TB cases

TABLE 2.10

The estimated burden of tuberculosis (TB) in India in 2013 as per the Global TB Report		
	Estimated incidence, 2013	Estimated number of deaths, 2013
All forms of TB	2.1 million (2.0–2.3 million) (rate 171)	0.24 milion* (0.15–0.35 million)
HIV-associated TB	0.12 million (0.1–0.14 million)	38,000 (31,000–44,000)
Multidrug-resistant TB	61,000 (47,000–76,000) amongst notified cases	26,000 (20,000–33,000) amongst notified cases

TB, tuberculosis; HIV, human immunodeficiency virus.
* Excluding deaths attributed to HIV/TB.

Source: World Health Organization Global Tuberculosis Report, 2014.

TABLE 2.11

Multidrug-resistant tuberculosis burden in India as per the survey carried out by Central Tuberculosis Division			
State (survey year)	Population	MDR among new cases	MDR among previously-Rx cases
Gujarat (2007–08)	56 million	2.4%	17.4%
Maharashtra (2008)	108 million	2.7%	14.0%
Andhra Pradesh (2009)	86 million	1.8%	11.8%

MDR, multidrug-resistant.

Estimated MDR-TB emerging annually from notified cases of pulmonary TB—64,000.

Population-based drug resistance surveillance (DRS) by the program in 3 states shows low MDR prevalence in new cases.

Extensively drug resistant among smear positive previously treated cases—0.5% (Gujarat DRS study) (~4,000 cases emerge annually).

is 1,000,000 (1,100,000–1,200,000), while the estimates of HIV positive incident TB cases in India is 90,000 (110,000–

TABLE 2.12

Drug-resistant tuberculosis burden in India as per reports from different duties in India

Study	setting	No. of MDR cases	No. of HIV positive	Prevalence of XDR-TB (%)	Reference
Mondal and Jain, 2007	Tertiary care centre, Lucknow	68	Not reported	5 (7.4)	Emerg infect Dis, 2007
Jain et al., 2007	Tertiary care centre, Mumbai	326	Not reported	36 (11)	ATS, abstract, 2007
Singh et al., 2007	Tertiary care centre, Delhi	12	All HIV-infected	4 (33.3)	AIDS, 2007
Thomas et al., 2007	Field trial, Chennai	66	Not reported	1 (1.5)	IJT, 2007
Sharma et al., 2009	AIIMS, New Delhi, tertiary care hospital	211	All HIV-negative	5 (2.4)	IJMR, 2009
Ramchandran et al., 2009	Gujarat, field study	216	Not reported	7 (3.1) All previously treated cases	IJTLD, 2009
Myneedu et al., 2011	LRS Institute, New Delhi	223	Not reported	45 (20.17%)	IJT, 2011

160,000). As per the WHO's Global TB Report of 2011, HIV prevalence among incident TB cases is estimated to be 3.3% (5–7.1%).

India has the third highest number of estimated people living with HIV in the world. According to the HIV estimations 2012, the estimated number of people living with HIV/AIDS in India was 20.89 lakh, with an estimated adult (15–49 age group) HIV prevalence of 0.27% in 2011. India has demonstrated an overall reduction of 57% in the annual new HIV infections among adult population from 2.74 lakh in 2000 to 1.16 lakh in 2011, reflecting the impact of various interventions and scaled-up prevention strategies under the National AIDS Control Program. The trend of annual AIDS deaths is showing a steady decline since roll out of the free antiretroviral therapy (ART) program in India in 2004; it is estimated that around 1.5 lakh lives have been saved due to ART till 2011.

Tuberculosis is one the important and detrimental opportunistic infection in patients living with HIV/AIDS. Human immunodeficiency virus among estimated incident TB patients is around 5.7% (4.8–6.6%). There are about 0.12 million (0.10–0.12 million) HIV-associated TB cases in India in 2013 and there were 38,000 (31,000–44,000) deaths in them. The mortality in the two groups (HIV-positive and negative) is shown in Figure 2.13.

Treatment outcomes in TB/HIV patients are not to that of non-HIV/TB patients. The outcome is shown in Table 2.13.

PEDIATRIC TUBERCULOSIS

Tuberculosis is among the top 10 causes of death among children worldwide; however, children with TB are given low priority in most national health programs and often neglected. There are about 1 million cases of pediatric TB globally, of

Epidemiology

which 75% occur in the 22 high burden countries. In low-burden countries, childhood TB constitutes approximately 5% of the TB caseload, in comparison to 20–40% in high burden

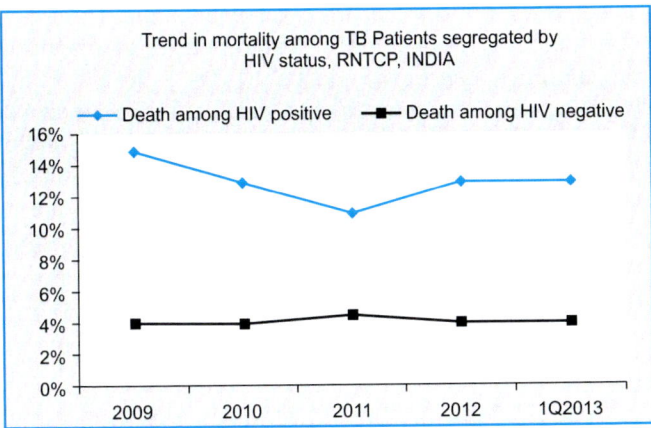

HIV, human immunodeficiency virus; RNTCP, Revised National Tuberculosis Control Program.

Figure 2.13 Mortality in human immunodeficiency virus positive and negative groups.

TABLE 2.13

Treatment outcome among all human immunodeficiency virus infected tuberculosis cases							
Type of cases	Total cases	Treatment success (%)	Died (%)	Failure (%)	TAD (%)	Transferred out (%)	Switched to category 4 (%)
New	30,394	79	13	1	5	1	1
Retreatment	13,553	71	14	2	8	3	2

TAD, treatment after default.

countries. Pediatric TB are estimated to occur every year accounting for 10–15% of all TB in the world; with more than 100,000 estimated deaths every year.

In India, there are about 400 million children who constitute about 34% of the total population. The extent of childhood TB in India is unknown due to diagnostic difficulties; it is estimated to be 10.2% of the total adult incidence. The maximum risk of a child getting TB is between 1–4 years when there is an increased risk of progression from infection to disease. Though MDR-TB and XDR-TB are documented among pediatric age group, there are no estimates of overall burden, chiefly because of diagnostic difficulties and exclusion of children in most of the drug resistance surveys. Trends in pediatric TB as reported to RNTCP in India is shown in the Figure 2.14.

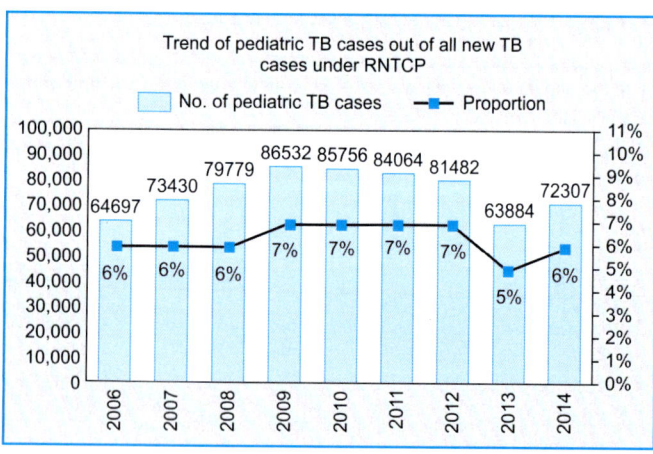

HIV, human immunodeficiency virus; RNTCP, Revised National Tuberculosis Control Program.

Figure 2.14 Pediatric tuberculosis in India as reported to Revised National Tuberculosis Control Program.

CURRENT TB SITUATION

Global Burden

As per the 2015 Global tuberculosis report released by WHO, in 2014, the TB situation has changed somehow as shown above for the year 2013. The same is shown in Table 2.14.

The distribution in different WHO regions is shown in Figure 2.15. The South-East Asia region has the highest burden (17%), followed by Western Pacific region with 17% of the global burden. Developed regions like the Americas and European regions the least number of 3% each. The five high burden countries of the world were India, China, Indonesia, Nigeria, and Pakistan. Of this 23% of the TB burden was only in India, followed by 10% each in Indonesia and China and

TABLE 2.14

Global burden of tuberculosis in 2014 (WHO report 2015)		
Tuberculosis	Estimated incidence, 2014	Estimated number of deaths, 2014
All forms	9.6 million (9.1–10 MIL) (5.4 M MALES; 3.2 M Women; 1.0 M Children) (rate133**)	1.1 million* (0.97–1.3 million)
HIV-associated	1.2 million (1.1–1.3million)	390,000 (350,000–430,000)
Multidrug resistant	480,000*** (360,000–600,000)	190,000 (120,000–260,000)
	300,000 (200,000 – 370,000) amongst notified cases	–

*Excluding deaths attributed to HIV/TB. **most cases occurring in Asia (56%) and Africa (29%). ***More than half of these patients were in India, China and the Russian Federation.

Source: WHO Global Tuberculosis Report 2015.

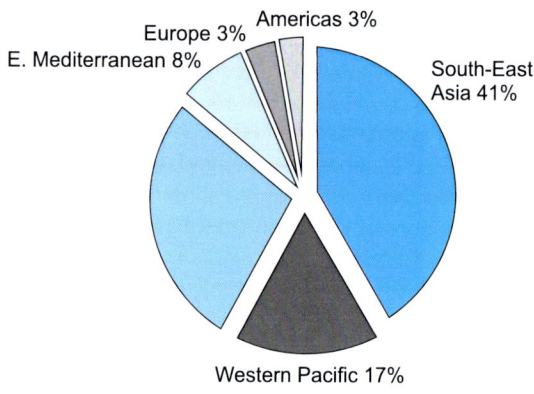

Figure 2:15 TB burden in different regions and countries in 2014.

5% each for Nigeria and Pakistan. Over half of these cases report to the private sector outside the National Tuberculosis Control Programs.

INDIAN SCENARIO IN 2014

The TB burden in India has also changed for the year 2014 as the WHO report-2015. The same has been shown in Table 2.15.

These data from India are estimates (guesstimates!) as reported to the program or calculated by the program. However, a vast majority of TB patients report to and are treated by the private sector and therefore, it is likely that these cases are not included in the calculation. To understand the true burden of the disease in the country, a group of investigators used a large, commercial data of sale and use of anti-TB drugs in the country over a period of two years. Then using a simulation model (Monte Carlo Simulation) they calculated the assumptions for

TABLE 2.15

Tuberculosis burden in India in 2014		
Tuberculosis	Estimated incidence, 2014	Estimated number of deaths, 2014
All forms	2.2 million (2.0–2.3 million) [Rate 167 (156–179)]	0.22 million* (0.15–0.35 million)
HIV-associated	0.11 million (0.096–0.120)	31,000 (25,000–38,000)
Multidrug resistant	New cases: 24,000 (21,000–29,000) Retreatment cases: 47,000 (35,000–59,000) **Total 71,000 (amongst notified cases)**	

*Excluding deaths attributed to HIV/TB. *Source:* WHO Global Tuberculosis Report 2015

average duration of tuberculosis treatment and accuracy of private diagnosis. There were 17.793 million patient-months (95% credible interval 16.709 million to 19.841 million) of anti-tuberculosis treatment in the private sector in 2014, twice as many as the public sector. If 40–60% of private-sector tuberculosis diagnoses are correct, and if private-sector tuberculosis treatment lasts on average 2–6 months, this implies that 1.19–5.34 million tuberculosis cases were treated in the private sector in 2014 alone. The midpoint of these ranges yields an estimate of 2.2 million cases, two to three times higher than currently assumed. These findings suggest that private sector in India is treating an enormous number of patients for tuberculosis, appreciably higher than has been previously recognized. Accordingly, there is a re-doubled need to address this burden and to strengthen surveillance. Tuberculosis burden estimates in India and worldwide require revision. A nation-wide survey will depict a correct picture.

> **KEY MESSAGE**
>
> ❑ The epidemiology of tuberculosis shows a wide variation world-wide. India has the highest number of TB cases. These estimates in different countries are based on reported cases through notifications and regional rather than national surveys. It is imperative to have a correct picture following correct epidemiological methods in all countries. However, it is clear that National TB Control Programs reduced the burden of the disease, and even some countries have achieved the MDG targets as envisaged.

SUGGESTED READINGS

1. Annual Report 2013-14. Department of AIDS Control, Ministry of Health & Family Welfare, Government of India.
2. Chadha VK, Agarwal SP, Kumar P, Chauhan LS, Kollapan C, Jaganath PS, et al. Annual risk of tuberculous infection in four defined zones of India: a comparative picture. Int J Tuberc Lung Dis. 2005;9:569-75.
3.. Dodd PJ, Gardiner E, Coghlan E, Seddon JA. Burden of childhood tuberculosis in 22 high-burden countries: a mathematical modeling study. Lancet Glob Health. 2014;2(8):e453-9.
4. Dye C, Bassili A, Bierrenbach AL, Broekmans JF, Chadha VK, Glaziou P, et al. Measuring tuberculosis burden, trends and the impact of control programmes. Lancet Infect Dis. 2008;8(4):233-43.
5. Dye C, Scheele S, Dolin P, Pathania V, Raviglione MC. Consensus statement. Global burden of tuberculosis: estimated incidence, prevalence, and mortality by country. WHO Global Surveillance and Monitoring Project. JAMA. 1999;282:677-8.
6. Dye C. Breaking a law: tuberculosis disobeys Stýblo's rule. Bull World Health Organization, 2008, 86:4.
7. Global Burden of Disease Study 2010. Lancet. 2012;380;9859.
8. Global Tuberculosis Report 2014. Available from: http://apps.who.int/iris/bitstream/10665/137094/1/9789241564809_eng.pdf.
9. Gopi PG, Prasad VV, Vasantha M, Subramani R, Tholkappian AS, Sargunan D, Narayanan PR. Annual risk of tuberculosis infection in Chennai city. Indian J Tuberc. 2008;55:157-61.

10. Indian Council of Medical Research. Tuberculosis in India - A Sample Survey (1955-58): Special Report Series No. 34, New Delhi.
11. Kumar A, Gupta D, Nagaraja SB, Singh V, Sethi GR, Prasad J. Updated National Guidelines for Pediatric Tuberculosis in India, 2012. Indian Pediatr. 2013;50: 301-30.
12. Marais BJ, Hesseling AC, Gie RP, Schaaf HS, Beyers N. The burden of childhood tuberculosis and the accuracy of routine surveillance data in a high burden setting. Int J Tuberc Lung Dis. 2006;10:259-63.
13. Murray CJ, Ortblad KF, Guinovart C, Lim SS, Wolock TM, Roberts DA, et al. Global, regional, and national incidence and mortality for HIV, tuberculosis, and malaria during 1990-2013: a systematic analysis for the Global Burden of Disease Study 2013. Lancet. 2014;pii:S0140-6736(14)60844-8.
14. Nelson LJ, Wells CD. Global epidemiology of childhood tuberculosis. Int J Tuberc Lung Dis. 2004;8:636-47.
15. Paramasivan CN, Venkataraman P. Drug resistance in tuberculosis in India. Ind J Med Res. 2004;120:377-86.
16. Swaminathan S, Rekha B. Pediatric Tuberculosis: Global Overview and Challenges. Clin Infect Dis. 2010;50(Suppl 3):S184-S194.
17. TB India 2015. Revised National TB Control Programme. Annual status report. Central TB Division, Government of India.
18. TB prevalence surveys: a handbook. World Health Organization: Geneva; 2011.
19. The Stop TB Strategy: building on and enhancing DOTS to meet the TB-related Millennium Development Goals. World Health Organization: Geneva; 2006.
20. Tiemersma EW, van der Werf MJ, Borgdorff MW, Williams BG, Nagelkerke NJ. Natural history of tuberculosis: duration and fatality of untreated pulmonary tuberculosis in HIV negative patients: a systematic review. PLoS One. 2011;6(4):e17601.
21. van Leth F, Van der Wert MJ, Borgdorff MW. Prevalence of tuberculous infection and incidence of tuberculosis: a re-assessment of the Styblo rule. Bulletin of the World Health Organization, 2008;86:20–26
22. WHO Calls Tuberculosis a Global Emergency. Los Angeles Times. 1993. Available from: www.//articles.latimes.com/1993.
23. Arinaminpathy N, Batra D, Khaparde S, Vualnam T, Maheshwari N, Sharma L, Nair SA, Dewan P.The number of privately treated tuberculosis cases in India: an estimation from drug sales data. Lancet Infect Dis. 2016; pii: S1473-3099(16):30259-6.

CHAPTER 3

The Organism

MORPHOLOGY AND BIOCHEMICAL CHARACTERISTICS

The tubercle bacillus, the causative organism for human tuberculosis (TB), was first discovered by Koch in 1882, and is known as *Mycobacterium tuberculosis*. The generic name *Mycobacterium* or the "fungus bacterium" was given because of the mould-like pellicle formed by the organism in liquid media. The Greek prefix *myco* means "fungus," alluding to the way mycobacteria have been observed to grow in a mold-like fashion on the surface of liquids when cultured. The bacillus is a member of the Mycobacteriaceae family. It is both acid- and alcohol-fast, obligate aerobe, nonspore-forming, and nonmotile bacillus, which grows and metabolizes rather slowly, and is resistant to a variety of deleterious influences. It grows best at 37°C. The organism is a facultative intracellular parasite, that is, it can grow within or outside of the cells. The bacillus is usually a slightly curved rod with parallel sides and rounded ends, ranging in size from (0.3 to 0.6) × 3 µm, straight, or slightly curved, occurring singly or in occasional strands. The organism stains uniformly or irregularly; often showing banded or beaded forms. Electron microscopy shows that mycobacteria possess a relatively thick cell wall, about 20 nm across. Mycobacteria are aerobic and nonmotile bacteria (except for the species *M. marinum*), characteristically acid fast. Mycobacteria have an outer membrane and do not have capsules, and most do not form endospores.

The distinguishing characteristic of all *Mycobacterium* species is that the cell wall is thicker than in many other bacteria, which is hydrophobic, waxy, and rich in mycolic acids/mycolates. The cell wall consists of the hydrophobic mycolate layer and a peptidoglycan layer held together by a polysaccharide, arabinogalactan. The cell wall makes a substantial contribution to the hardness of this genus. Many *Mycobacterium* species adapt readily to growth on very simple substrates, using ammonia or amino acids as nitrogen sources and glycerol as a carbon source in the presence of mineral salts. Optimum growth temperatures vary widely according to the species and range from 25°C to over 50°C. Mycobacteria are classical acid-fast organisms. Stains used in evaluation of tissue specimens or microbiological specimens include Fite's stain, Ziehl-Neelsen stain, and Kinyoun stain. Mycobacteria appear phenotypically most closely to members like *Nocardia*, *Rhodococcus,* and *Corynebacterium*. The cell wall is neither truly Gram negative nor positive. In addition, they are naturally resistant to a number of antibiotics that disrupt cell wall biosynthesis such as penicillin. Due to their unique cell wall, they can survive long exposure to acids, alkalis, detergents, oxidative bursts, lysis by complement, and many antibiotics. Most mycobacteria are susceptible to the antibiotics clarithromycin and rifamycin, but antibiotic-resistant strains have emerged. As with other bacterial pathogens, surface and secreted proteins of *M. tuberculosis* contribute significantly to the virulence of this organism. There is an increasing list of extracytoplasmic proteins proven to have a function in the virulence of *M. tuberculosis*. Mycobacteria can be classified into several major groups for purpose of diagnosis and treatment: *M. tuberculosis* complex(*M. tuberculosis*, *M. bovis*, *M. africanum*, and *M. microti)*, which can cause TB; *M. leprae*, which causes Hansen's disease or leprosy; and nontuberculous mycobacteria are all the other mycobacteria, which can cause pulmonary disease resembling TB, lymphadenitis, skin disease, or disseminated disease. Mycosides are phenolic alcohols (such as phenolphthiocerol) that were shown to be components of *Mycobacterium* glycolipids which are termed glycosides of phenolphthiocerol dimycocerosate. There are 18 and 20 carbon atoms in mycosides A and B, respectively. Comparative analyses of mycobacterial genomes have identified several conserved indels and signature proteins that are uniquely found in all sequenced species from the genus *Mycobacterium*. Additionally, 14 proteins are found only in the species from the genera *Mycobacterium* and *Nocardia*, suggesting that these two genera are closely related. The position of *M. tuberculosis* in the genus is shown in Figure 3.1.

Mycobacterium tuberculosis complex (MTBC) involves *M. tuberculosis*, *M. bovis*, *M. bovis* BCG, *M. africanum*, *M. microti, M. cannetii, M. caprae,* and *M. pinnipedii* and cause human and animal TB. The causative organism for TB is the *M. tuberculosis,* which is one of the most widely spread disease causing mycobacteriosis in humans. The MTBC species are closely related taxonomic group of bacteria contributing to about 100% chromosomal homology between each other. The *M. tuberculosis* genome is about 4.4 Mbp and contains 0.01–0.3% synonymic nucleotide polymorphisms. Of the many Mycobacteria, only *M. tuberculosis*, *M. bovis,* and *M. africanum* are recognized as tubercle bacilli. Mycobacteria vary enormously in their metabolic activities, nutritional requirements, and rate of growth. The basic requirements of mycobacterial growth *in vitro* are carbon, nitrogen, oxygen, phosphorous, sulfur, iron, magnesium, sodium, potassium, and various other trace elements.

The Organism

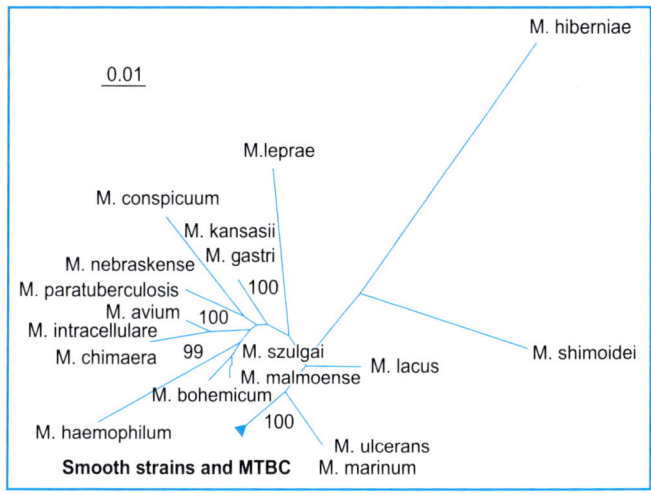

Figure 3.1 Phylogenetic position of the tubercle bacilli within the genus *Mycobacterium*. The blue triangle corresponds to tubercle bacilli sequences that are identical or differing by a single nucleotide. The sequences of the genus *Mycobacterium* that matched most closely to those of *M. tuberculosis* were retrieved from the BIBI database and aligned with those obtained for 17 smooth and *M. tuberculosis* complex strains. The unrooted neighbor-joining tree is based on 1,325 aligned nucleotide positions of the 16S ribosomal ribonucleic acid gene. The scale gives the pairwise distances after Jukes-Cantor correction. Bootstrap support values higher than 90% are indicated at the nodes.

Many identification tests based on metabolic activities include niacin production and arylsulfatase, phosphatase, catalase, and reductase activity. The organism is susceptible to heat, which is taken advantage of in the process of pasteurization. They have higher resistance to acids, alkalis, and chemical disinfectants. Mycobacteria are destroyed by disinfectants like phenol, hypochlorite, or glutaraldehyde solution. Ethylene oxide and formaldehyde are suitable for sterilization of fiber optic bronchoscopes except that the gases have poor penetration to kill bacilli embedded in sputum. The organisms are rapidly killed by acetone, propanol, and 70% ethanol, which are useful for disinfection of skin, clinical thermometers, and bench tops. Formaldehyde is suitable for disinfection of safety cabinets. Mycobacteria are resistant to drying and survive for weeks or months on inanimate objects. The low permeability of the mycobacterial cell wall is thought to contribute to resistance of mycobacteria to antibiotics and chemotherapeutic agents. The nature of mycolic acid plays a crucial role in determining the fluidity and permeability of mycobacterial cell wall. The cell wall is the most complex among all the bacteria. A particular characteristic is the high lipid content (60% of the cell wall weight). It contains up to 60% lipids as against some 20% for the lipid-rich cell wall of Gram-negative organisms. The genus is distinguished by characteristic antigenic patterns and mycolic acid structures. The G + C content of deoxyribonucleic acid are 66–72 mol/dL.

The lipids render the surface of *M. tuberculosis* hydrophobic. Of the many fatty acids, cord factor (trehalose 6,6'-dimycolate), cardiolipin, mycolic acid, Wax D, and sulfatides are the important one for its pathogenetic characteristics. The organism also contains carbohydrates and protein. The cell wall structure has been depicted in Figure 3.2. It has several layers.

The principal feature of the cell wall is the dense palisade of characteristic long chain fatty acids—the mycolic acids. Wax D, is a complex chloroform soluble molecule composed of a mycolic acid linked through a small arabinogalactan to a fragment of murein. Units of Wax D may arise by autolysis or may be building blocks from which the cell wall is constructed. Lipids of mycobacteria are unique to the genus. Many of them are long-chain fatty acids modified by the presence of unsaturated bonds. Some of them are the mycolic acid, mycoserosic acid,

The Organism

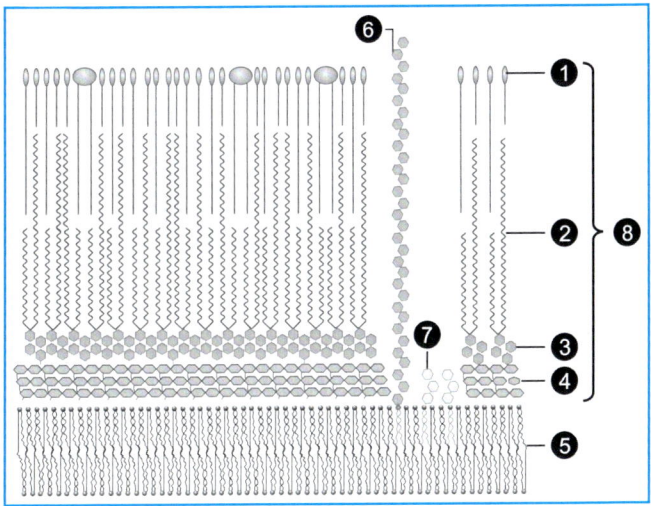

Figure 3.2 Mycobacterial cell wall. 1, outer lipids; 2, mycolic acid; 3, polysaccharides (arabinogalactan); 4, peptidoglycan; 5, plasma membrane; 6, lipoarabinomannan; 7, phosphatidylinositol mannoside; 8, cell wall skeleton. *(For color version, see Plate 2)*

phthienoic acid, and tuberculostearic acid. The mycolic acids are long-chain lipids having an alkyl chain attached to the methylene group. They contain around 60–90 carbon atoms. The size of these lipids is an important criterion of the genera. Two important classes of lipid contain the disaccharide trehalose: sulfolipids and trehalose dimycolates, also known as "cord factors". Sulfolipids are strongly acidic compounds consisting of mycoserosic acid covalently linked to trehalose sulfate. Sulfolipid is a major determinant of virulence of the organism. Cord factor, 6,6'-dimycoloyl-a,a'-D-trehalose, consists of two mycolic acids linked to trehalose. The name was given with the erroneous belief that it is responsible for the characteristic "serpentine cords" of *M. tuberculosis*. It was also erroneously believed that this factor is related to virulence. However, it has a toxic action, the relevance of which to pathogenesis is not clear. Mycosides are heterogeneous group biologically important species or strain-specific cell surface lipids.

The lipids are responsible for many characteristics like:
- Acid fastness
- Slow growth
- Resistance to detergents
- Antibiotic resistance
- Antigenicity
- Clumping.

Protein secretion systems are now considered as the main virulence factors of pathogenic bacteria. *M. tuberculosis* has five type 7 secretion systems (ESX1-5). The best characterized of these is ESX1, which is missing in the attenuated *M. bovis* vaccine strain Bacille Calmette-Guerin, and is required for the full virulence of *M. tuberculosis*. Another group of proteins known to play an important role in pathogenesis are those under the control of the dormancy survival regulon, which controls expression of more than 50 genes responsible for the *M. tuberculosis* hypoxic response.

Mycobacterial antigens are broadly classified as:
- Cytoplasmic (soluble) or cell wall lipid-bound (insoluble)
- According to their chemical structure (carbohydrate or protein)
- By their distribution within the genus.
- Up to 15–90 lines of soluble antigens can be demonstrable depending on the method of testing applied.

These soluble antigens are further divided into four major groups:
- Group I or those common to all mycobacteria (also found in *Nocardia*, *Corynebacterium*, and *Listeria*)
- Group II occurring in slowly growing species

TABLE 3.1

Mutation rates of *Mycobacterium tuberculosis* to different drugs	
Drugs	Mutation rate
Rifampicin	2.3×10^{-10}
Isoniazid	2.6×10^{-8}
Ethambutol	1.0×10^{-7}
Streptomycin	3.0×10^{-9}

- Group III occurring in rapidly growing species
- Group IV are those unique to each individual species.

Study of genomes of mycobacterial chromosomes revealed that they have molecular weights of (2.5–5.55 kDa) and *M. tuberculosis* being at the lower end of the spectrum. Mutations occur naturally at a low frequency to various antituberculous drugs. The mutation rates of *M. tuberculosis* to the commonly used antituberculous drugs vary and the spontaneous mutation rates are shown in Table 3.1.

Several different repetitive elements are known to be present in the *M. tuberculosis* genome of which IS6110 is the most widely studied element. It is specific for the *M. tuberculosis* complex and has been used extensively as a genetic target in the identification and epidemiologic mapping of *M. tuberculosis*. Mycobacteriophages lyse the mycobacteria. Phage typing of *M. tuberculosis* shows four types designated as A, B, C, and I. Most strains are of type A, I, or B; type C is very rare. Most, but not all, phage type I are of the guinea-pig-attenuated South Indian variant of *M. tuberculosis*.

Staining Characteristics

Tubercle bacilli are described as Gram positive although they resist decolorization by alcohol after staining with basic dyes. When stained with carbol fuchsin by the Ziehl-Neelsen method or by fluorescent dyes, auramine O/rhodamine, they resist decolorization by 20% sulfuric acid and absolute alcohol for 10 minutes (acid and alcohol fast). This acid-fastness may be either due to the presence of an unsaponifiable wax (mycolic acid) in the bacillus or due to a semipermeable membrane around the cell. Beaded or barred forms are frequently seen in *M.tuberculosis*, but *M. bovis* invariably stains uniformly.

The bacilli grow slowly, the generation time being 14–15 hours. Colonies appear in about 2 weeks and may sometimes take up to 8 weeks. The optimum growth temperature is about 37°C and growth is inhibited below 25°C and above 40°C. The optimum pH is 6.4–7.0; *M. tuberculosis* is an obligate aerobe, while *M. bovis* is microphillic on primary isolation, becoming aerobic on subculture. *Mycobacterium tuberculosis* grows luxuriously in culture (eugenic) compared to *M. bovis,* which grows sparsely (dysgonic). Addition of 0.5% glycerol improves the growth of *M. tuberculosis* while this causes inhibition or no effect on the growth of *M. bovis*. Sodium pyruvate helps the growth of both. Human tubercle bacilli do not grow in the presence of P-nitrobenzoic acid, unlike other slow growing nonchromogens.

Genomic Structure of *Mycobacterium tuberculosis*

The complete genome sequencing was done in 1998 and comprises 4,411,529 base pairs, contains around 4,000 genes, and has a very high guanine + cytosine content that is reflected in the biased amino acid content of the proteins. *Mycobacterium tuberculosis* differs radically from other bacteria in that a very large portion of its coding capacity is devoted to the production of enzymes involved in lipolysis, and to two new families of glycine-rich proteins with a repetitive structure that may represent a source of antigenic variation. Annotation of the *M. tuberculosis* genome shows

The Organism

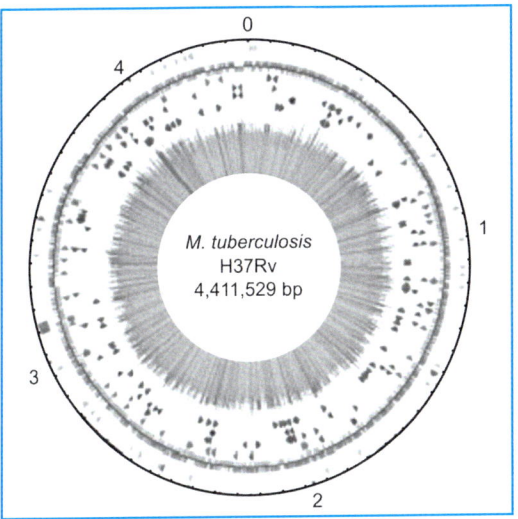

Figure 3.3 Circular map of the chromosome of *M. tuberculosis* H37Rv. *(For color version, see Plate 3)*

that this bacterium has some unique features. Over 200 genes are annotated as encoding enzymes for the metabolism of fatty acids, comprising 6% of the total. The circular map of the chromosome and the electron photomicrograph of *M. tuberculosis* H37Rv are depicted in Figures 3.3 and 3.4.

Molecular Epidemiology of Tuberculosis

There are three widely used genotyping tools to differentiate *M. tuberculosis* strains; namely, IS6110 restriction fragment length polymorphism, spacer oligotyping (Spoligotyping), and mycobacterial interspersed repeat units-variable number of tandem repeats. A new prospect towards molecular epidemiology was introduced with the development of whole genome sequencing and the next generation sequencing methods, where

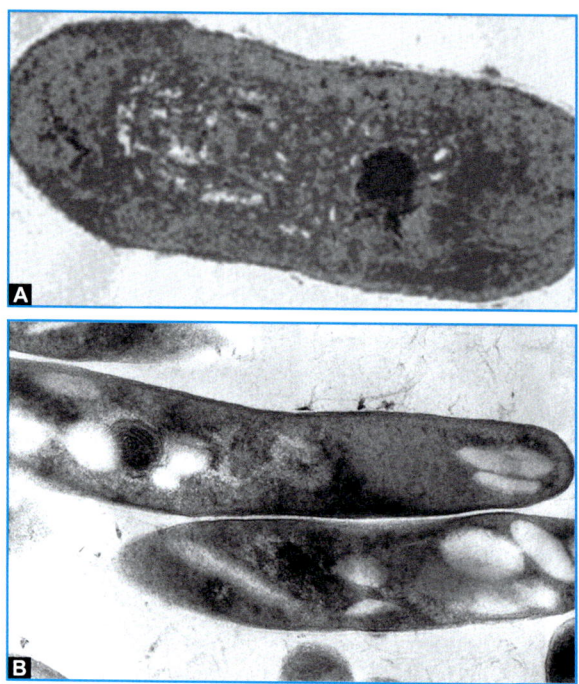

Figure 3.4 Electron micrograph of *Mycobacterium tuberculosis*. *(For color version, see Plate 4)*

the entire genome is sequenced. Next generation sequencing is also found to be useful in identifying single nucleotide polymorphisms, comparative genomics, and also various aspects about transmission dynamics. These techniques enable the identification of mycobacterial strains and also facilitate the study of their phylogenetic and evolutionary traits.

The main human-infecting species have been classified into seven spoligotypes:
- Type 1 contains the East African-Indian and some Manu (Indian) strains

- Type 2 is the Beijing group
- Type 3 consists of the Central Asian strains
- Type 4 of the Ghana and Haarlem, Latin America-Mediterranean and X strains
- Types 5 and 6 correspond to *M. africanum* and are observed predominantly and at very high frequency in West Africa
- Type 7 has been isolated from the Horn of Africa.

Other species of this complex belong to a number of spoligotypes and do not normally infect humans. Types 2 and 3 are more closely related to each other than to the other types. Types 5 and 6 are most closely aligned with the species that do not normally infect humans. Type 3 has been divided into two clades: CAS-Kili (found in Tanzania) and CAS-Delhi (found in India and Saudi Arabia). The clinical relevance of strain variation among *M. tuberculosis* isolates has long been a matter of dispute.

> **KEY MESSAGE**
>
> ❏ Tuberculosis is caused by a micro-organism—the *Mycobacterium tuberculosis*. The organism was discovered by Robert Koch in the year 1882. Since then many of its morphological and molecular characteristics have been described. Various virulent factors causing the disease have also been identified. The use of electron microscope has further delineated its ultrastructure. The cell-wall of the Mycobacteria is the most important component and is, perhaps responsible for its virulence.

SUGGESTED READINGS

1. Bates JH, Mitchison DA. Geographic distribution of bacteriophage types of Mycobacterium tuberculosis. Am Rev Res Dis. 1969;100:189-93.
2. Brennan PJ. Structure, function, and biogenesis of the cell wall of Mycobacterium tuberculosis. Tuberculosis. 2003;83:91-7.

3. Cole ST, Brosch R, Parkhill J, Garnier T, Churcher C, Harris D, et al. Deciphering the biology of Mycobacterium tuberculosis from the complete genome sequence. Nature. 1998;393:537-44.
4. Daniel TM, Janicki BW. Mycobacterial antigens: a review of their isolation, chemistry, and immunological properties. Microbiol Rev. 1978;42:84-113.
5. Desikan S, Narayanan S. genetic markers, genotyping methods and next generation sequencing in mycobacterium tuberculos. Indian J Med Res. 2015;141:761-74.
6. Gomez JE, Chen JM, Bishai WR. Sigma factors of Mycobacterium tuberculosis. Tubercle Lung Dis. 1997;78:175-83.
7. Goren MB. Mycobacterial lipids: selected topics. Bacteriol Rev. 1972;36:33-64.
8. Horsburgh CR Jr. Tuberculosis. Eur Respir Rev. 2014;23:36-9.
9. Jones WD Jr. Geographic distribution of phage types among cultures of Mycobacterium tuberculosis. II. Cultures from India and South Africa. Am Rev Respir Dis. 1990;142:1000.
10. Minnikin DE. In Ratledge C, Stanford JL, editors. The biology of the mycobacteria. Academic Press: New York; 1982. *p. 95*.
11. Parish T, Brown A, editors. Mycobacterium: genomics and molecular biology. Caister Academic Press: London; 2009.
12. van Crevel R, Nelwan RHH, de Lenne W, Veeraragu Y, van der Zanden AG, Amin Z, et al. Mycobacterium tuberculosis Beijing genotype strains associated with febrile response to treatment. Emerg Infect Dis. 2001;7:1-4.

CHAPTER 4
Pathogenesis of Tuberculosis

INTRODUCTION

When people with active pulmonary tuberculosis (TB) cough, sneeze, speak, sing, or spit, they expel infectious aerosol droplets 0.5–5.0 μm in diameter. A single sneeze can release up to 40,000 droplets. Most infections are asymptomatic and latent, but about 1 in 10 latent infections eventually progresses to active disease which, if left untreated, kills more than 50% of those so infected. The infectious dose of TB is very low. Inhalation of fewer than 10 bacteria may cause an infection. People with prolonged, frequent, or close contact with people with TB are particularly at high risk of becoming infected, with 22% infection rate.

A person with active but untreated TB may infect at least 10–15 other people per year. Transmission only occurs from people with active TB and not with latent infection. Probability of transmission depends upon several factors: number of infectious droplets expelled by the carrier, effectiveness of ventilation, duration of exposure, virulence of the *M. tuberculosis* strain, and level of immunity in the uninfected person. Person-to-person transmission can be circumvented by effectively segregating those with active (overt) TB and putting them on anti-TB drug regimens. After about 2 weeks of effective treatment, subjects with nonresistant active infections generally do not remain contagious to others. If someone does become infected, it typically takes three to four weeks before the newly infected person becomes infectious enough to transmit the disease to others.

About 90% of those infected with *M. tuberculosis* have asymptomatic, latent TB infections (LTBI), with only a 5–10% lifetime chance of progress to overt, active TB disease. Human immunodeficiency virus (HIV) increases the risk of developing active TB to nearly 10% a year. A number of risk factors increase the chance of development of active TB in the host (Box 4.1).

Genetic susceptibility to TB is thought to be a contributor. Certain populations appear to have a high degree of vulnerability to TB—Eskimos in North America, Yanomami Indians in the Brazilian Amazon, and Black populations in the

BOX 4.1

Risk factors for development of tuberculosis

- Human immunodeficiency virus/acquired immune deficiency syndrome
- Other immunosuppressed states
  - Corticosteroids and other immunosuppressants
  - Antimitotic drugs
  - Infleximab
- Renal failure, cirrhosis of liver
- Malignancies, particularly lymphomas and leukemias
- Silicosis/anthracosis
- Partial gastrectomy
- Healthcare workers
- Diabetes mellitus
- Smoking
- Malnutrition
- Indoor air pollution
- Overcrowding
- Close family contacts
- Slums, jail inmates
- Intravenous drug abusers
- Shelter homes
- Extremes of age
- Alcoholism
- Genetic predisposition (?)
- Pregnancy
- Old history of tuberculosis
- Psychiatry disorders

United States. A substantial percentage of individuals recover even without treatment. Several polymorphisms in the human *NRAMP1* gene have been identified, and population-based studies have identified increased relative risk for moving from latent infection to active disease associated with certain polymorphisms.

Toll-like receptor 2 (TLR2) G2258A is associated with increased TB risk, especially in Asians and Europeans. Toll-like receptor 1 G1805T is associated with increased TB in Africans and American Hispanics. Toll-like receptor 6 C745T is associated with decreased TB risk. Several other genes and gene families, including those for vitamin D receptors and the components of interferon-γ (INF-γ) signaling pathways possibly have role in susceptibility to TB. The tubercle bacillus (1–5 μm) enters the lower respiratory tract. Larger sized droplets are efficiently excluded by physical barriers of the nasopharynx and upper respiratory tract or removed by the mucociliary blanket. After inhalation, the droplet nucleus is carried down the bronchial tree and implants in a respiratory bronchiole or alveolus.

Fewer than 10% of organisms will reach the respiratory bronchioles and alveoli. Whether or not an inhaled tubercle bacillus establishes an infection in the lung will depend on both the bacterial virulence and the inherent microbicidal ability of the alveolar macrophage that ingests it. If the bacillus is able to survive initial defenses, it can multiply within the alveolar macrophage. The organism grows slowly, dividing approximately every 25–32 hours within the macrophage. It has no known endotoxins or exotoxins; therefore, there is no immediate host response to infection.

The organisms grow for 2–12 weeks until they reach 10^3–10^4 in number, which is sufficient to elicit a cellular immune response that can be detected by tuberculin skin test.

Clinic Consult Pulmonology: Tuberculosis

Before the development of cellular immunity, tubercle bacilli spread via the lymphatics to the hilar lymph nodes and thence through the bloodstream to more distant sites. Certain organs and tissues are notably resistant to subsequent multiplication of these bacilli. The bone marrow, liver, and spleen are almost always seeded with mycobacteria, but uncontrolled multiplication of the bacteria in these sites is exceptional. Organisms deposited in the upper lung zones, kidneys, bones, and brain may find environments that favor their growth, and numerous bacterial divisions may occur before specific cellular immunity develops and limits multiplication.

The respiratory bronchial epithelium is remarkably resistant to infection by *M. tuberculosis*, although virulent mycobacteria are cytotoxic for alveolar type II cells. The bronchial epithelium produces antimicrobial peptides with a wide spectrum of activity. Tuberculosis infection begins when the mycobacteria reach the pulmonary alveoli, where they invade and replicate within endosomes of alveolar macrophages. The primary site of infection in the lungs, known as the "*Ghon focus*", is generally located in either in the upper part of the lower lobe, or the lower part of the upper lobe. Tuberculosis of the lungs may also occur via infection from the blood stream. This is known as a "Simon focus" and is typically found in the apex of the lung. This hematogenous transmission can also spread infection to more distant sites, such as peripheral lymph nodes, the kidneys, the brain, and the bones. All parts of the body can be affected by the disease, though for unknown reasons it rarely affects the heart, skeletal muscles, pancreas, or thyroid.

Once organisms have made their way into the lung, they can have four potential effects:

1. The initial host response can be completely effective and kill all bacilli and the patient has no chance of developing TB at any time in the future

Pathogenesis of Tuberculosis

2. The organisms can begin to multiply and grow immediately after infection, causing clinical primary TB
3. Bacilli may become dormant and never cause disease at all, the patient will have latent infection, manifest only by a positive tuberculin skin test
4. The latent organisms can eventually begin to grow, with resultant clinical disease, known as reactivation TB.

The possible fate of invading *M. tuberculosis* is shown in Figure 4.1.

Currently, most TB infections are initiated through the respiratory route of exposure only, as milk products are generally pasteurized. Prior to the acquired immune deficiency syndrome epidemic, 85% of new TB cases were pulmonary. Different forms of the disease (extrapulmonary) usually arise from dissemination of the bacilli from infected lungs.

Tuberculosis, in many cases, follows a general pattern as described by Wallgren, who divided the progression and resolution of the disease into four stages:

1. In the first stage, dating from 3 to 8 weeks after *M. tuberculosis* contained in inhaled aerosols becomes implanted in alveoli, the bacteria are disseminated by the lymphatic circulation to regional lymph nodes in the lung,

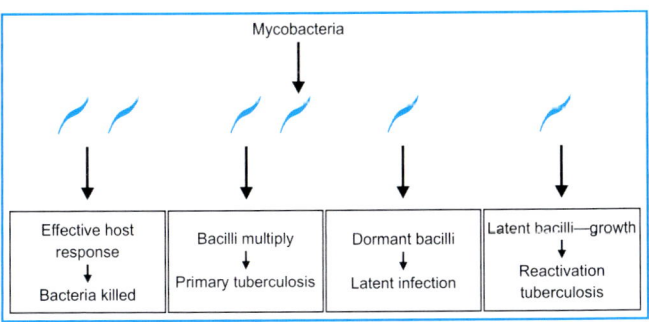

Figure 4.1 Possible fate of inhaled mycobacteria in the lungs.

forming the so-called primary or Ghon complex. At this time, conversion to tuberculin reactivity occurs

2. The second stage, lasting about 3 months, is marked by hematogenous circulation of bacteria to many organs including other parts of the lung; at this time in some individuals, acute and sometimes fatal disease can occur in the form of tuberculous meningitis or miliary (disseminated) TB

3. Pleurisy can occur during the third stage, lasting 3–7 months and causing severe chest pain, but this stage can be delayed for up to 2 years. It is thought that this condition is caused by either hematogenous dissemination or the release of bacteria into the pleural space from subpleural concentrations of bacteria in the lung. The free bacteria or their components are thought to interact with sensitized CD4 T lymphocytes that are attracted and then proliferate and release inflammatory cytokines

4. The last stage or resolution of the primary complex, where the disease does not progress, may take up to 3 years. In this stage, more slowly developing extrapulmonary lesions, e.g., those in bones and joints, frequently presenting as chronic back pain, can appear in some individuals.

The Wallgren time table is shown in Table 4.2–4.4.

The possible organ involvement has been depicted in form of sketch diagram in Figure 4.2.

Most humans who are infected with TB do not exhibit progression of the disease. One-third of the exposed HIV-negative individuals become infected, and of this number 3–5% develops in the first year. An additional 3–5% of those infected develop TB later in their lives. It is thought that most adult TB in non-HIV-infected patients is caused by reactivation of preexisting infection. Human immunodeficiency virus-positive persons infected with *M. tuberculosis* have a 50% chance of developing reactivation (post-primary) TB at

Pathogenesis of Tuberculosis

TABLE 4.2

Stage	Duration	Features
1	3–8 weeks	The primary complex develops; conversion occurs (tuberculin positivity)
2	About 3 months	Life-threatening forms of disease due to hematogenous dissemination like tuberculous meningitis and miliary tuberculosis
3	About 3–4 months	Tuberculous pleurisy may be the result of either hematogenous spread or direct spread from an enlarging primary focus
4	Up to 3 years	This stage lasts until the primary complex resolves; extrapulmonary tuberculosis may evolve more slowly particularly the bones and joints
5	Up to 12 years	Genitourinary tuberculosis may develop as a late manifestation of primary tuberculosis

TABLE 4.3

Organ	Time course
Pulmonary tuberculosis	Within a few months after primary infection
Miliary and meningeal tuberculosis	2–6 months
Lymph node tuberculosis	3–9 months
Bones and joints	Several years
Renal and genital tuberculosis	May take over a decade

Pulmonary lesions occurring as a result of reactivation of a dormant focus previously established in the body takes a number of years after primary infection.

some time in their lives. These individuals and others who are immunosuppressed can also be newly infected with *M. tuberculosis* and in many cases show rapid progression to active disease. Adult TB, whether resulting from activation

TABLE 4.4

Possible time table for development of clinical tuberculosis in different organs after primary infection		
Type of tuberculosis	*Time after infection*	*Comments*
Miliary tuberculosis and tuberculous meningitis	Within 6 months	Common in children under the age of 5 years; meningitis may be a terminal event in the cryptic miliary disease in elderly
Pleural effusion	6–12 months	Common in young adults
Progressive primary or post-primary disease	1–2 years	Common at puberty; the primary disease can progress with increasing infiltration and cavitation
Skeletal tuberculosis	1–5 years	Common in spines
Genitourinary and cutaneous tuberculosis	5–15 years	–

or new infection in HIV-infected patients, is almost always pulmonary and is associated with differing degrees of lung involvement and damage, notably necrosis, cavitation, and bleeding.

Tuberculosis is classified as one of the granulomatous inflammatory diseases. Macrophages, T lymphocytes, B lymphocytes, and fibroblasts are among the cells that aggregate to form granulomas, with lymphocytes surrounding the infected macrophages. The granuloma prevents dissemination of the mycobacteria and provides a local environment for interaction of cells of the immune system. Bacteria inside the granuloma can become dormant, resulting in latent infection. Another feature of the granulomas is the development of abnormal cell death (apoptysis/necrosis) in the center of tubercles. To the naked eye, this has the texture of soft, white cheese and is termed as

Pathogenesis of Tuberculosis

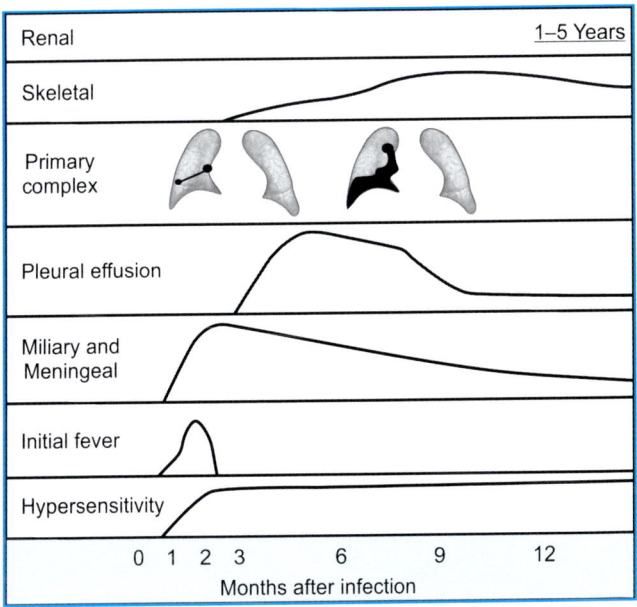

Figure 4.2 Fate of primary complex.

caseous necrosis. If TB bacteria gain entry to the bloodstream from an area of damaged tissue, they can spread throughout the body and set up many foci of infection, all appearing as tiny, white tubercles in the tissues. This severe form of TB disease, most common in young children and those with HIV, is called "miliary tuberculosis". People with this disseminated TB have a high fatality rate even with treatment (about 30%).

In many people, the infection waxes and wanes. Tissue destruction and necrosis are often balanced by healing and fibrosis. Affected tissue is replaced by scarring and cavities filled with caseous necrotic material. During active disease, some of these cavities are joined to the air passages bronchi and this material can be coughed up. It contains living bacteria, and so can spread the infection. Treatment with appropriate drugs kills bacteria and allows healing to take place. Upon cure, affected areas are eventually replaced by scar tissue. The bacilli resist the innate immune response mediated by alveolar macrophages in 20–50% of persons exposed. Active multiplication within the macrophages continue infecting nearby cells and activating the immune response. Host immunity plays an important role in the host-pathogen interaction occurring in persons exposed to *M. tuberculosis*. The host mounts a cell mediated immune response that leads to a cellular infiltration (granuloma). In 90–95% of cases, this host immune response inhibits bacterial multiplication, controlling the growth of the infectious agent and leading to a latent infection (latent TB).

Latent TB is clinically silent, with no outward signs or symptoms of disease, and is characterized by the presence of a specific cell mediated immune response specific for *M. tuberculosis*, classically highlighted by Mantoux test or a positive INF-γ release assay (IGRA) test. People with latent TB have a 5–10% chance of developing active TB during their lifetime as host immune response cannot completely eradicate the bacteria *in vivo* and that the immune response itself does not provide a lifetime protection against the emergence of active disease. In 5–10% of cases, the host immune response fails to control primary infection and it is the host response itself that is responsible for the extensive tissue damage and necrosis that is the hallmark of active TB in immune-competent patients. Latent TB infection represents a positive skin reaction to tuberculin but had no symptoms of TB, pulmonary or extrapulmonary. In contrast to patients with active TB disease, latently infected individuals are not infectious and chest radiographs have no abnormalities or signs of healed TB disease.

There is a great variability in the course of *M. tuberculosis* infections among humans. Some persons remain uninfected, which is evidenced by a negative tuberculin skin test and/or IGRA for LTBI, despite prolonged exposure to infectious TB cases. In most people, a primary *M. tuberculosis* infection induces the development of specific acquired cell mediated immunity inhibiting the growth of mycobacteria without their eradication. In such individuals, TB bacilli persist in a dormant state. The risk of reactivation of latent TB for immunocompetent subjects is in the order of 10% in a lifetime. Upon infection, *M. tuberculosis* primarily stimulates type 1 [T helper 1 (Th1)] cytokine reaction that is driven by the CD4+ T cells. Key cytokines in this reaction are interferon-γ (IFN-γ) and tumor necrosis factor-α (TNF-α), which synergize to activate microbicidal effector mechanisms in human macrophages. This is the base of the delayed type hypersensitivity caused by *M. tuberculosis* antigens and this phenomenon has been used for more than a century to identify *M. tuberculosis*-infected subjects by the tuberculin skin test. Cell mediated immunity is the major component of host defense against TB. In resistant individuals, the control of *M. tuberculosis* infection relies on the development of a Th1 immune response. This type of response involves the participation of a number of cells that include resident alveolar macrophages, dendritic cells, T lymphocytes (TCD4+, TCD8+, Tγδ), and release of proinflammatory cytokines, IFN-γ, interleukin (IL)-2, IL-12, IL-18, TNF-α, and a number of chemokines [IL-8, monocyte chemoattractant protein-1, macrophage inflammatory proteins-1α, etc.]. All of them play an important role in the recruitment of additional cells to the infection site for the formation of granuloma that contains and kills TB bacilli, but also provides a long-time niche needed for LTBI. Humoral response may not be relevant for protection. Macrophage is capable of inhibiting growth of bacillus through phagocytosis, and participating in a broader context of cellular immunity through the process of antigen presentation and recruitment of T-lymphocytes. The march of events after the mycobacterial infection between the organism and the macrophage involves a series of steps that decides in which way the result will be.

Phagocytosisis engulfs the invading microbe through a membrane-bound tight vacuole that is created when number of pseudopods surround the bacterium and fuse distally. Creation of this vacuole, or phagosome, is accompanied by binding of the organisms to the phagocyte through complement receptors CR1, CR3, and CR4, as well as mannose receptors (MRs) and other cell surface receptor molecules. Complement activation plays an important role in this process. There also may be differences between specific binding mechanisms for virulent and relatively avirulent strains of mycobacteria. In the process, the initiation of agent-host interaction in the lungs (the infectious process) can be divided into the "early" and "late" events. In the early events, resident macrophages, but possibly alveolar epithelial type II pneumocytes and dendritic cells play a very important role. Surfactant protein A, can enhance the binding and uptake of M. tuberculosis by upregulating MR activity. Surfactant protein D inhibits phagocytosis of M. tuberculosis by blocking mannosyl oligosaccharide residues on the bacterial cell surface, which prevents M. tuberculosis interaction with MRs on the macrophage cell surface. Cholesterol in cell plasma membranes is thought to be important for this process. The human TLR2 also plays a role in M. tuberculosis uptake. Phagosome-lysosome fusion, creates hostile environment that includes acidic pH, reactive oxygen intermediates (ROIs), lysosomal enzymes, and toxic peptides. Reactive nitrogen intermediates (RNIs) produced by activated mouse macrophages are major elements in antimicrobial activity. Reactive nitrogen intermediates are the most significant weapon against virulent mycobacteria in mouse macrophages and resistance to RNIs among various strains of M. tuberculosis correlates with virulence. The presence of RNIs in human macrophages and their potential role in disease has been the subject of controversy, but the alveolar macrophages of a majority of TB-infected patients exhibit inducible nitric oxide synthase activity. Since most macrophage killing of bacteria occurs in the phagolysosome, intracellular pathogens have evolved many ways to avoid this hostile vacuolar microenvironment. Phagosome-lysosome fusion without acidification also occurs due to exclusion of proton adenosine triphosphatases (ATPase) from the mycobacterial phagosome. Opsonization directs bacterial binding to Fc receptors. Role of Ca^{2+} signaling is another possibility in the pathogenesis. There is a decrease in the expression of major histocompatibility complex (MHC) class I proteins and in the MHC-II presentation of bacterial antigens induced by presence of secreted or surface-exposed *M. tuberculosis* 19 kDa lipoprotein, by interaction with TLR2.

LATER EVENTS

There is much less information on how the bacterium survives and grows during later stages of infection in the lung. It is known that infected macrophages in the lung, through their production of chemokines, attract inactivated monocytes, lymphocytes, and neutrophils, none of which kill the bacteria very efficiently. Then, granulomatous focal lesions composed of macrophage-derived giant cells and lymphocytes begin to form. This process is generally an effective means of containing the spread of the bacteria.

As cellular immunity develops, macrophages loaded-bacilli are killed. This results in formation of the caseous center of the granuloma, surrounded by a cellular zone of fibroblasts, lymphocytes, and blood-derived monocytes. *Mycobacterium tuberculosis* bacilli are unable to multiply within this caseous tissue due to acidic pH, the low availability of oxygen, and the presence of toxic fatty acids. Some organisms may remain dormant but alive for decades. The strength of the host cellular immune response determines whether an infection is arrested here or progresses to the next stages. This enclosed infection is referred to as latent or persistent TB and can persist throughout a person's life in an asymptomatic and nontransmissible state.

In persons with efficient cell mediated immunity, the infection may be arrested permanently at this point. The granulomas subsequently heal, leaving small fibrous and calcified lesions. If an infected person cannot control the initial infection in the lung or if a latently infected person's immune system becomes weakened, the granuloma center becomes liquefied and serves as a rich medium in which the bacteria can replicate in an uncontrolled manner. At this point, viable *M. tuberculosis* can escape from the granuloma and spread within the lungs (active pulmonary TB) and even to other tissues via the lymphatic system and the blood (miliary or extra-pulmonary TB). In response to invading mycobacteria, the host innate immune system recognizes the pathogen through innate receptors. It produces appropriate effector proteins, including cytokines. These innate signals activate or regulate autophagic pathways during infection. Vitamin D and functional vitamin D receptor signaling are critical in the activation of autophagic defenses.

FATE OF MYCOBACTERIUM TUBERCULOSIS AFTER ENGULFMENT

Pathogenic bacteria are killed by a variety of mechanisms: phagosome-lysosome fusion, generation of ROIs, and generation of RNIs, particularly nitric oxide. Mycobacteria protect themselves by producing ammonia, which could inhibit the phagosome-lysosome fusion and, also by alkalinizing the intralysosomal contents, thus diminishing the potency of the fusion complex. Sulfatides (derivatives of trehalose 2-sulfate, a glycolipid produced by *M. tuberculosis*) also inhibit phagosome-lysosome fusion. The exact role of these potential "escape" mechanisms in the pathogenesis of human disease is uncertain.

Many other biochemical events like excluding proton-ATPase from the phagosome, and arrest of mycobacterial phagosome maturation at rab-7, can also take active role in the ultimate outcome. Once inside the macrophage, *M. tuberculosis* can be killed by several other different mechanisms through a host of complicated interactions, mediated by cytokines, between lymphocytes and phagocytes. The ability of mycobacteria to evade killing by either reactive oxygen or nitrogen species may be a crucial step in the establishment of the latent state of infection.

Some of the unique features of *M. tuberculosis* that are contributory to its pathogenesis is the annotation of the genome. Over 200 genes are annotated as encoding enzymes for the metabolism of fatty acids, comprising 6% of the total. Some genes have also been identified as being upregulated during infection. *Mycobacterium tuberculosis* has developed strategies to maintain redox homeostasis, including mechanisms to regulate endogenous nitric oxide and carbon monoxide levels to maintain redox homeostasis, including mechanisms to regulate endogenous nitric oxide and carbon monoxide levels. *Mycobacterium tuberculosis* regulatory metalloproteins are sensitive to exogenous stresses attributed to changes in the levels of gaseous molecules (i.e., molecular oxygen, carbon monoxide, and nitric oxide) to elicit an intracellular response. Recent developments have highlighted on the subfamily of Whi proteins, redox sensing WhiB-like proteins that contain iron-sulfur clusters, sigma factors, and their cognate antisigma factors of which some are zinc-regulated, and the dormany survival regulon DosS/DosT-DosR heme sensory system. Cytotoxic T-lymphocytes can ingest macrophages that have engulfed mycobacteria. They can also secrete small proteins such as TIA-1, a cytoplasmic molecule that has been shown to be associated with apoptosis (programed cell death).

The interaction of macrophages with other effector cells occurs in a milieu of both cytokines and chemokines. These molecules serve both to attract other inflammatory effector cells such as lymphocytes and to activate them. An important chemokine in the mycobacterial host-pathogen interaction appears to be IL-8. They have the ability to recruit neutrophils, T-lymphocytes, and basophils. Development of granuloma is mediated partly by the intercellular adhesion molecule-1, a surface molecule that is upregulated by *M. tuberculosis* or lipoarabinomannan. This upregulation is mediated by increased gene expression directly by mycobacteria and can be amplified by the cytokines TNF-α, IL-6, and INF-γ. The differentiated macrophage-epithelioid cells produce extracellular matrix proteins (i.e., osteopontin and fibronectin), which provide a cellular anchor.

Mycobacteria are also capable of inducing caseation necrosis tribute to this process, caseation necrosis occurs in animal models lacking the 55 kDa TNF receptor. Recently, it is demonstrated that lymphangioleiomyomatosis could upregulate interstitial collagenase gene expression in peripheral blood monocytes; in addition, it is shown that the 92 kDa gelatinase (matrix metalloproteinase 9) gene is also induced. These two proteins of the extracellular matrix can digest collagens I, III, and IV as well as other matrix proteins. The matrix metalloproteinases 9 gene was strikingly upregulated in bronchoalveolar lavage cells recovered from patients with cavitary TB.

Pathogenesis of Tuberculosis

HOST IMMUNE RESPONSE

Human system evades or protects itself against microorganisms through innate (inherited) or acquired immunity. *Mycobacterium tuberculosis* has acquired the ability to establish latent or progressive infection and persist even in the presence of a fully functioning immune system. The ability of *M. tuberculosis* to avoid immune mediated clearance is likely to reflect a highly evolved and coordinated program of immune evasion strategies, including some that interfere with antigen presentation to prevent or alter the quality of T cell responses. There are multiple mechanisms by which *M. tuberculosis* actively inhibit, subvert, or otherwise modulate antigen presentation by MHC class I, class II, and CD1 molecules.

Toll-like receptors play an essential role in the recognition of *M. tuberculosis* components by macrophages and dendritic cells, resulting in not only activation of innate immunity but also development of antigen specific adaptive immunity.

Induction of early death of the infected cells may be one of the strategies of host defense against *M. tuberculosis* because macrophages go into apoptosis upon infection with *M. tuberculosis*, resulting in suppression of the intracellular replication.

Interferon-γ plays an important role in protection. In the process, the effects of proinflammatory (TNF) and antiinflammatory (IL-10) cytokines play important roles on the spectrum of phagocyte populations (macrophages and dendritic cells) in the lung and lymph node. Tumor necrosis factor is a major mediator of recruitment of phagocytes to the lungs. In contrast, IL-10 is a factor in balancing the dominant macrophage phenotype in lymph nodes and lung. The intricate interaction of the various components of the cellular immune system occurs in a fluid environment containing a wide variety of chemokines and cytokines, and it is likely that the precise balance of these various factors has a large impact on the body's ability to successfully contain infection.

In vitro and animal studies complemented by human studies using bronchoalveolar lavage from patients with TB and from control subjects has enhanced our understanding that may be useful for therapy. The immune response in TB are of two categories: immunity or protection and delayed hypersensitivity and tissue damage, although in some there may not be any response. The former protects and the later causes damage.

The immune response is under genetic control. The macrophages process the antigenic determinants of tubercle bacilli and transfer them along with the MHC antigen to the antigen specific T cells (CD4 and CD8). CD4 cells recognize antigens when presented along with class II MHC antigen coded in human leukocyte antigen (HLA)-D genes. CD8 cells recognize antigen in association with class I MHC antigen coded in HLA-A and HLA-B genes. Which of the MHC antigen is to be presented in the macrophage is genetically determined and thus varies from person to person. This decides the type of immune response whether it will be protective thus eliminating the bacteria or a delayed hypersensitivity reaction leading to necrosis, tissue damage, and clinical disease. Once the antigen-MHC complex is attached to the T cells, they undergo stimulation and clonal multiplication. A wide range of reactions is set into motion depending on the genetic makeup of the host like induction or suppression of immunity, activation of macrophages for bacteriolysis, production of memory cells for immediate encounter in case the bacteria reappear again, delayed hypersensitivity reaction causing granulomatous inflammation, necrosis, tissue damage, and development of tuberculin test response.

Some believe that CD4 and CD8 cells have different subsets with an initiating immunity and the other hypersensitivity reaction determined genetically. CD4 cell subset CD4-Th1 helps immunity by producing IL-2 and IFN-γ and CD4-Th2 helps delayed hypersensitivity through secretion of IL-4 and IL-5.

Pathogenesis of Tuberculosis

Class II (HLA-DR and HLA-DR2) genes are associated with the development of smear positive pulmonary TB. These genes may determine the cells, Th1 or Th2, to which mycobacterial antigen is to be presented. Both specific and nonspecific immunity can be transferred to a healthy animal only by lymphocyte transfer and not of macrophages or serum of an immune animal. In thymectomized animals treated with antilymphocyte serum, the cell mediated immune response vanishes or diminishes.

Delayed hypersensitivity and tissue damage follows activation of the T helper cells (CD4) by antigens that secrete INF-γ and other lymphokines that activate macrophages. The TNF-γ converts inactive vitamin D3 to active calcitriol or active-vitamin D3. Calcitriol triggers release of TNF, which in turn activates many phagocytic cells and helps in formation of granuloma. In others, it kills the sensitized cells leading to necrosis. Some products of T cells may sensitize cells to toxic effects of TNF and this depends on the particular subset of T helper cells involved.

British Medical Research Council's TB vaccines trial shows that greatest risk of disease following primary infection is within the first two years. About 54% develop disease within a year of infection and 78% within 2 years. Rates for subsequent years are given in Table 4.5.

TABLE 4.5

Rates for subsequent years	
1st year	54%
2nd year	24%
3rd year	9%
4th year	5%
5th and 6th year	3%
7th and 8th year	3%
9th + years	1%

Clinic Consult Pulmonology: Tuberculosis

Possible clinical course from exposure to disease is shown in Figure 4.3. Risk factors include HIV/AIDS, other immunosuppressive states, and immunity status.

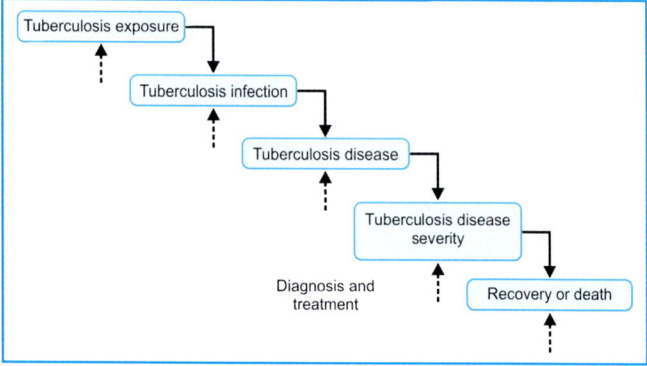

HIV, human immunodeficiency virus; AIDS, acquired immune deficiency syndrome.

Figure 4.3 Possible clinical course from exposure to disease.

KEY MESSAGE

- Even if the human being is exposed to tubercle bacilli, only a few of them develop disease (about 5–10% life-time risk). However, in immunosuppressed states like HIV infection, immunosupressant drug use (steroids, cyclophosphamide, cancer chemotherapy etc), certain occupations, certain malignant diseases, and organ dysfunction states, the chances of developing the disease increases. By and large it is a self limiting infection without progression to disease in a majority of cases. Certain other factors also increases the risk of tuberculosis. Almost any organ of the body can be affected by tuberculosis. The infection can also remain dormant for a long period of time and with certain conditions can be reactivated.

SUGGESTED READINGS

1. Abdallah AM, Gey van Pittius NC, Champion PA, Cox J, Luirink J, Vandenbroucke-Grauls CM, et al. Type VII secretion--mycobacteria show the way. Nat Rev Microbiol. 2007;5:883-91.
2. Bhatt K, Salgame P. Host innate immune response to Mycobacterium tuberculosis. J Clin Immunol. 2007;4:347-62.
3. Bradfute SB, Castillo EF, Arko-Mensah J, Chauhan S, Jiang S, Mandell M, et al. Autophagy as an immune effector against tuberculosis. Curr Opin Microbiol. 2013;16:355-65.
4. Chen K, Kolls JK. T cell-mediated host immune defenses in the lung. Annu Rev Immunol. 2013;31:605-33.
5. Cobat A, Orlova M, Barrera LF, Schurr E. Host genomics and control of tuberculosis infection. Public Health Genomics. 2013;16:44-9.
6. Co DO, Hogan LH, Kim SI, Sandor M. Mycobacterial granulomas: keys to a long-lasting host-pathogen relationship. Clin Immunol. 2004;113:130-6.
7. Coelho Filho JC, Takenami I, Arruda S. Revisiting the Rich's formula: an update about granulomas in human tuberculosis. Braz J Infect Dis. 2013;17:234-8.
8. Cole E, Cook C. Characterization of infectious aerosols in health care facilities: an aid to effective engineering controls and preventive strategies. Am J Infect Control. 1998;26:453-64.
9. Dannenberg AM Jr. Roles of cytotoxic delayed-type hypersensitivity and macrophage-activating cell-mediated immunity in the pathogenesis of tuberculosis. Immunobiology. 1994;191:461-73.
10. Druszczynska M, Kowalewicz M, Marek Fol K, WŁOdarczyk M, Rudnckaw W. Latent M. tuberculosis infection—pathogenesis, diagnosis, treatment and prevention strategies. Polish J Microbiol. 2012;61:3-10.
11. Fenton MJ, Vermeulen MW. Immunopathology of tuberculosis: roles of macrophages and monocytes. Infect Immun. 1996;64:683-90.
12. Forrellad MA, Klepp LI, Gioffré A, Sabio y García J, Morbidoni HR, de la Paz Santangelo M, et al. Virulence factors of the Mycobacterium tuberculosis complex. Virulence. 2013;4:3-66.
13. Fox GJ, Barry SE, Britton WJ, Marks GB. Contact investigation for tuberculosis: a systematic review and meta-analysis. Eur Respir J. 2013;41:140-56.

14. Israel H, Hetherington H, Ord J. A study of tuberculosis among 44 students of nursing. JAMA. 1941;117:461-73.
15. Jagirdar J, ZagZag D. Pathology and insights into pathogenesis of tuberculosis. In: Rom WN, Garay S, editors. Tuberculosis. Little, Brown and Co.: Boston, MA; 1996.
16. Kawamura I. Protective immunity against Mycobacterium tuberculosis. Kekkaku. 2006;81:687-91.
17. Koch R. A further communication on a remedy for tuberculosis. BMJ 1890;2:1193-5.
18. Law KF, Jagirdar J, Weiden MD, Bodkin M, Rom WN. Tuberculosis in HIV-positive patients: cellular response and immune activation in the lung. Am J Respir Crit Care Med. 1996;153:1377-84.
19. Lienhardt C, Fielding K, Sillah JS, Bah B, Gustafson P, Warndorff D, et al. Investigation of the risk factors for tuberculosis: a case-control study in three countries in West Africa. Int J Epidemiol. 2005;34:914-23.
20. Lin PL, Flynn JL. Understanding latent tuberculosis: a moving target. J Immunol. 2010;185:15-22.
21. Mcdonough KA, Kress Y, Bloom BR. Pathogenesis of tuberculosis: Interaction of Mycobacterium tuberculosis with macrophages. Infect Immun. 1993;61:2763-73.
22. Nau GJ, Guilfoile P, Chupp GL, Berman JS, Kim SJ, Kornfeld H, et al. A chemoattractant cytokine associated with granulomas in tuberculosis and silicosis. Proc Natl Acad Sci USA. 1997;94:6414-9.
23. Nicas M, Nazaroff WW, Hubbard A. Toward understanding the risk of secondary airborne infection: emission of respirable pathogens. J Occup Environ Hyg. 2005;2:143-54.
24. Pope AS, Philip E, Sartwell PE, Zacks D. Development of tuberculosis in infected children. Am J Public Health Nations Health. 1939;29:1318-25.
25. Rathored J, Sharma SK, Singh B, Banavaliker JN, Sreenivas V, Srivastava AK, etc. Risk and outcome of multidrug-resistant tuberculosis: vitamin D receptor polymorphisms and serum 25(OH) D. Int J Tuberc Lung Dis. 2012;16:1522-8.
26. Riley L. Phagocytosis of M. tuberculosis. In: Rom W, Garay S, editors Tuberculosis. Little, Brown, Boston, MA 1996;281-9.
27. Schluger NW, Rom WN. The host immune response to tuberculosis. Am J Respir Crit Care Med. 1998;157:679-91.

28. Schluger NW. The pathogenesis of tuberculosis the first one hundred (and twenty-three) years. Am J Respir Cell Mol Biol. 2005;32:251-6.
29. Slight SR, Khader SA. Chemokines shape the immune responses to tuberculosis. Cytokine Growth Factor Rev. 2013;24:105-13.
30. Smith I. Mycobacterium tuberculosis pathogenesis and molecular determinants of virulence. Clin Microbiol Rev. 2003;16:463-96.
31. Spector WG, Lykke AW. The cellular evolution of inflammatory granulomata. J Pathol Bacteriol. 1966;92:163-7.
32. Stead WW, Senner JW, Reddick WT, Lofgren JP. Racial differences in susceptibility to infection by Mycobacterium tuberculosis. N Engl J Med. 1990;322:422-7.
33. Stein CM, Zalwango S, Malone LL, Won S, Mayanja-Kizza H, Mugerwa RD, et al. Genome scan of M. tuberculosis infection and disease in Ugandans. PLoS One. 2008;3:e4094.
34. van Crevel R, Ottenhoff TH, van der Meer JW. Innate immunity to Mycobacterium tuberculosis. Clin Microbiol Rev. 2002;15:294-309.
35. Wagner R. Clemens von Pirquet, discoverer of the concept of allergy. Bull NY Acad Med. 1964;40:229-35.
36. Wallgren A. The time table of tuberculosis. Tubercle. 1938;29:245-51.
37. Wells W. Airborne contagion and air hygiene. Harvard University Press: Cambridge, MA; 1955.

CHAPTER 5

Pathology of Tuberculosis

PRIMARY TUBERCULOSIS

The bacilli will be deposited in the alveoli and a small patch of caseous bronchopneumonia develops; this encapsulates later. This is the "primary focus" or "Ghon's focus". The regional lymph node is soon involved and together they are called the "primary complex" (parenchymal lesion + lymph node). The bacilli reach the lymph node within less than an hour of reaching the lung and often the blood. Attraction of neutrophils and macrophages to the site of infection leads on to cascade of events. The primary infection can develop at any lung zone, but is common in the lower part of the upper lobe or in the upper part of the lower lobe, chiefly in the right; seldom found in the apex. The lesion is situated closer to pleura. Other lymph nodes become involved by lymphatic spread both upwards toward the neck and downwards to the abdomen. The first implant can occur anywhere in the lung, and the cavitary lesion is often located in the apical region of the lungs. Even if the primary implant can occur anywhere in the lungs, for the progression from infection to disease, the tubercle bacilli must gain access to the vulnerable regions in the apex of the lungs.

In areas of the world where there is low risk of infection with tubercle bacilli, low incidence of vaccination or

Pathology of Tuberculosis

sensitization to environmental mycobacteria, or high incidence of high virulent isolates, the virulent tubercle bacilli reach the vulnerable region via a bacillemia during the first infection. In areas of a high risk of infection, high incidence of vaccination or sensitization to environmental mycobacteria, or a high incidence of low virulent isolates, the tubercle bacilli reach the vulnerable region via the airways, which requires repeated episodes of infection.

The primary foci may follow one of the following consequences:
- Most foci become quiescent and calcify
- Some of the calcified foci, especially those in the lymph nodes may recrudesce at a later stage and become the source of progressive pulmonary/extrapulmonary tuberculosis (TB)
- A primary lesion may also, soon after formation, becomes the center of progressive disease either by liquefaction and subsequent eruption into the (i) bronchi, (ii) vessels, or (iii) by transmission of bacilli to the hilar nodes and then to the blood stream.

The fate of a primary focus is summarized in Figure 5.1.

Early development of primary focus starts with the multiplication of bacilli during the first few days in the alveoli. Epithelioid cell formation appears as the first recognizable, characteristic tubercular lesion called "tubercle" 6–8 days after inhalation. The epithelioid cells are macrophages, which develop pale foamy cytoplasms rich in lipid and crowd together. Some mononuclear cells fuse to form the multinucleated or Langhans giant cells. The center of the lesion liquefies causing caseation necrosis, the characteristic of a tubercular granuloma. The small foci enlarge and undergo caseation necrosis. This becomes arrested soon and a capsule is formed in the collapsed tissue around the focus, which mainly consists of fibrous tissue.

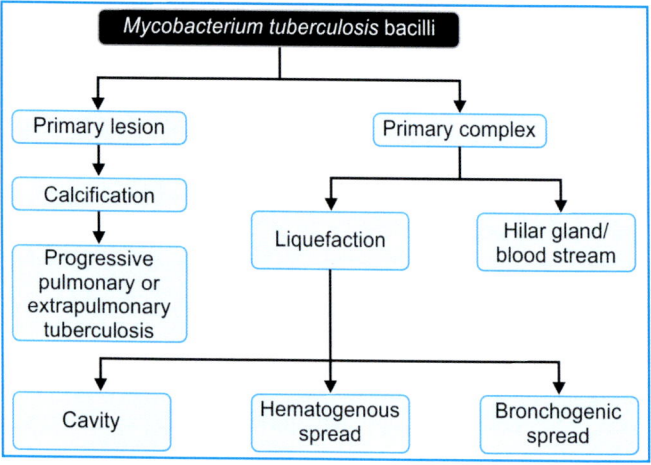

Figure 5.1 Possible course of a primary focus.

Three to six weeks after inhalation, the primary focus is fully developed and sometimes calcified in the center. After lymphocytic demarcation of the central caseous area, recrudescence may cause further fresh caseation outside the ring of lymphocytes. The calcified lesions may contain acid-fast bacilli on histologic section.

Granuloma is the typical pathological change which is a structural organization of different types of immune cells, macrophages, T cells, B cells, dendritic cells, neutrophils, natural killer cells, and a fibroblast which is formed in response to pulmonary inflammation resulting from the stimulation of host cells with mycobacterial antigens (Figure 5.2). Granuloma is initiated by resident macrophages that phagocytose bacilli and release proinflammatory cytokines, such as tumor necrosis factor-α, and additional cells are recruited. Macrophages undergo differentiation into epithelioid cells or they fuse to form

Pathology of Tuberculosis

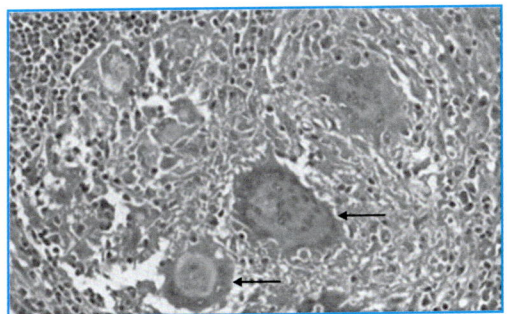

Figure 5.2 Granuloma and Langhan's giant cells.
(For color version, see Plate 4)

multinucleated giant cells within the granuloma. Various cells mentioned above that take part in the reaction, are surrounded by a rim of lymphocytes including CD4 T cells of adaptive immune response. The bactericidal capacity of macrophages is enhanced by the release of interferon-γ. At a later stage, a tight cover of fibroblasts encloses the granuloma. The adapted cell mediated immune response and proper formation of granuloma determine the outcome of *M. tuberculosis* infection (Figure 5.3). Sarcoidosis is a condition where one can find granulomas. However in this condition, the granulomas are noncaseating, compact and naked and at times one may get inclusion bodies; whereas those due to tuberculosis are caseating with necrosis, they are ill-formed with intense inflammation. The two differentiating granuloas are seen in Figure 5.4.

REACTIVATED OR POST-PRIMARY TUBERCULOSIS

The primary lesion sometimes progresses and the pathologic changes will then be similar to those seen in reactivation TB. The main difference between the primary infection and

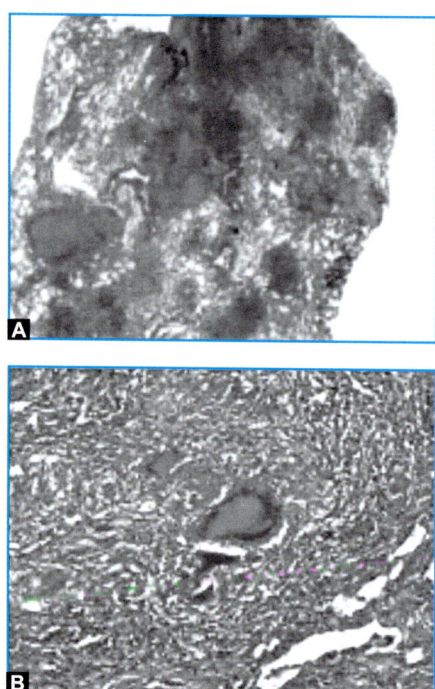

Figure 5.3 Tuberculous granuloma. *(For color version, see Plate 5)*

reactivation is that, while in former the involvement of the regional lymph node is an essential component of pathology, in the latter, regional lymph node is not necessarily involved. Due to an early bacteremia following the formation of a primary lesion in the hilar glands, the bacilli are carried by the lymphatics to the right heart and then again into the lungs. These foci are called "Simon's foci." These are essentially the Post-primary lesions commonly seen in chronic disseminated and extrapulmonary TB, both on radiology and at autopsy. They also occur in a large number of primarily infected

Pathology of Tuberculosis

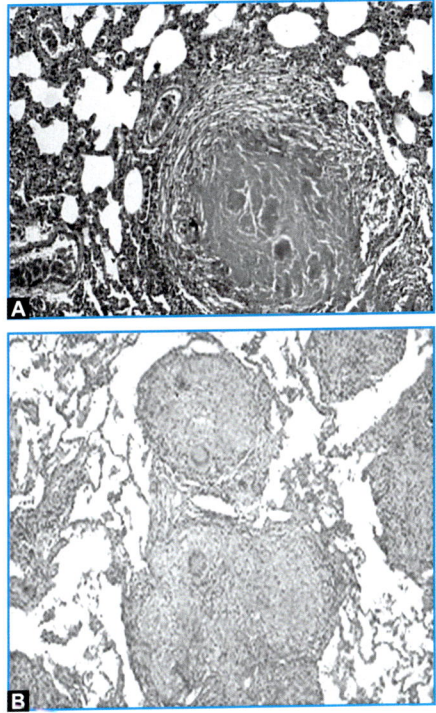

Figure 5.4 Granuloma of tuberculosis and sarcoidosis. *(For color version, see Plate 6)*

individuals as accidental findings. In case of primary intestinal TB, small calcified nodules may sometimes be seen in liver, which originate in a direct hematogenous transmission of the bacilli to the liver from the intestine via the portal vein.

Reactivated pulmonary TB is often seen in the upper lung zones and is limited in extent most frequently to the posterior segment of the upper lobe or apex of the lower lobe. The high alveolar partial pressure of oxygen in the upper zones relative to the other lung zones due to high ventilation-perfusion

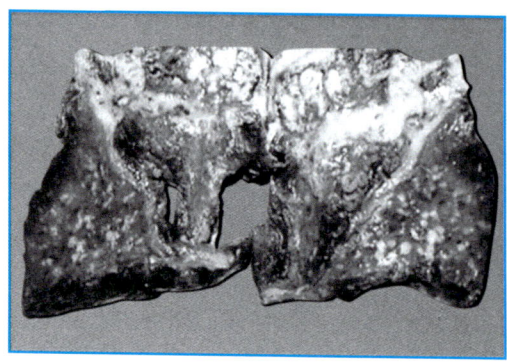

Figure 5.5 Fibrocaseous tuberculosis with cavitation (post-primary tuberculosis). *(For color version, see Plate 6)*

predisposes to reactivation at these sites. Softening and liquefaction of the caseous material, which may discharge, into a bronchus with resultant cavity formation, follow proliferation of tubercle bacilli in the caseous center (Figure 5.5).

While 10^4 bacilli per gram are found in caseous tissue, up to 10^9 organisms may be harbored within a single cavity. Fibrous tissue forms around the periphery of such tuberculous lesions but is usually incapable of limiting extension of the tuberculous process. Hemorrhages may result from extension of the caseous process into vessels within the cavity walls.

Spread of caseous and liquefied material through the bronchial tree may disseminate the infection to other lung zones with or without the development of vigorous inflammatory exudates or tuberculous pneumonia. This type of reaction is sometimes due to a hypersensitivity reaction to tubercular protein released by the dead bacilli, and is called "epituberculosis."

Rupture of a caseous pulmonary focus into a blood vessel may result in miliary TB with the formation of multiple

0.5–2 mm tuberculous foci in the lung and in other organs of the body. Encroachment on the bronchi of pulmonary or lymph node caseous material may give rise to tuberculous bronchitis. Rupture of caseous glands into trachea or major bronchi causes collapse of lung or even sudden death by suffocation particularly in young children. Vasculitis secondary to TB affecting the affected vessels like pulmonary or cerebral is not an uncommon finding.

Post-primary lesions can be divided into four main types:

1. Nodular type
    - Small
    - Large
2. Fibrocaseous type
    - With cavity
    - Without cavity
3. Miliary lesions
4. Mixed nodular and fibrocaseous lesions.

All these lesions represent active tuberculous pathology meaning necrosis of varying extent with scanty to profuse epithelioid and giant cell reaction in the surrounding area.

Healed tuberculous lesions may also present as small nodules but are almost always located in the subpleural region which are completely fibrosed or show mixtures of calcification, ossification, and carbon pigment deposition. The frequency of active tuberculous disease was about 17% in autopsy series. Nodular lesions comprise a little more than half of all active cases in the lungs, the fibrocaseous variety about 45%, and the miliary almost 2%. The small nodule is 1 cm or less in diameter, has a relatively thick fibrocollagenous capsule which isolates the central area of necrosis from the almost normal appearing lung outside. The population of epithelioid and giant cells in these lesions is generally small and scattered. In contrast, large nodules which are greater than 1 cm in diameter but still relatively well delineated from the neighboring lung parenchyma by a thin, irregular, and relatively inconspicuous capsule, shows much more prominent epithelioid cells and giant cell reaction surrounding a large area of central necrosis. Satellite small nodules may be present in the periphery of these large nodules. Special stains on these small nodules reveal preservation of the alveolar framework in the central necrotic area indicating that the basic process is one of the lobular pneumonia which has gone on to necrosis. The larger nodules can be found in close association with fibrocaseous lesion indicating a transition from the former to the latter.

The fibrocaseous and military lesions are self-explanatory. The frequency of demonstration of tubercle bacilli in the tissue section varies from 7, 29, and 75% in the small, large, and fibrocaseous type nodules, respectively. The corresponding figures in the microbiologic studies are 9, 36, and 77%, respectively. There is a good correlation between pathology and microbiology. Small nodules, which appear insignificant and inconspicuous, act as reservoirs, without producing any clinical symptom. It is potentially dangerous and under altered conditions like lowered host immunity, can break through the barrier producing more extensive tuberculous disease.

The evolution of disease will depend largely on the immune status of the individual at the time of invasion. In a nonimmune individual, an initial lobular pneumonia would most frequently lead on to necrosis, which in turn would produce the characteristic primary complex (Figure 5.6).

Rarely, the lobular pneumonia undergoes complete resolution to produce a scar. A primary complex would generally heal with fibrosis and calcification because of the development of immunity and will produce a healed nodule. Very rarely, when the immune competence is inadequate, progressive primary disease would lead to a larger complex, florid TB, extrapulmonary spread, or disseminated military TB.

Pathology of Tuberculosis

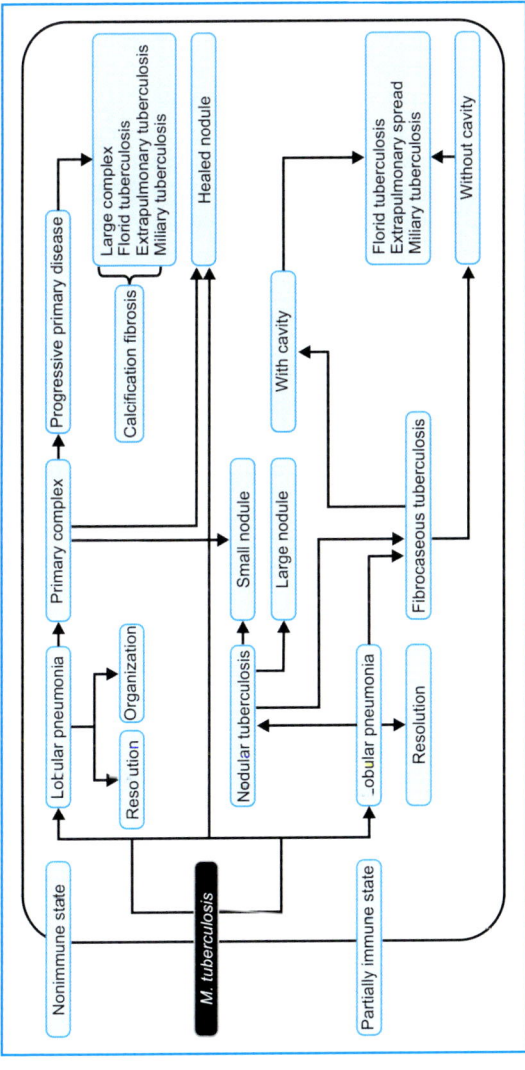

Figure 5.6 Natural history of clinical tuberculosis.

In a partially immune individual, the initial lobular pneumonia would most frequently lead on to either a nodular form or a fibrocaseous type of TB. Very rarely, complete resolution would occur. The nodular lesion is usually the small nodular type, which may completely heal and like the primary complex, may lead to a healed nodule. Some of the nodules, large or small, may progress to form fibrocaseous TB. A primary complex can convert into an active nodule. Fibrocaseous form of the disease frequently cavitates but a small proportion may continue as such. These fibrocaseous lesions are caused by low immunity status of the individual and might lead to extensive form of the disease in the lungs, to extrapulmonary sites, and disseminated miliary TB. Figure 5.6 represents the natural history of pulmonary TB.

The progression of the granulomatous response in mice infected with *M. tuberculosis* follows five distinct immuno-pathologic stages:
1. Mild scattered
2. Moderate
3. Moderate granulomatous
4. Moderately coalescing
5. Extensive.

KEY MESSAGE

❑ Following infection with *M. tuberculosis*, the course of tuberculosis is variable. Either it will lead to a stable and healed lesion or can remain quiscent for a varying period of time till it will progress to disease depending upon the host immunity; or it may be a progressive disease. The disease either called as a primary or post-primary lesion. Demonstration of caseating granuloma is the hall mark of tubercular pathology; however it needs to be differentiated from other granulomatous lesions like sarcoidosis. Granuloma of both these diseases, of course, are different.

SI, Sandor M. Mycobacterial granulomas: host-pathogen relationship. Clin Immunol.

protective immune response to Mycobacterium r Opin Immunol. 1995;7:512-6.

hun SI, Doran HM, Wilson P. Association between ical diagnosis of tuberculosis and microbiological ubercle Lung Dis. 1994;75:75-9.

WI. Granulomatous hypersensitivity. Prog Allergy. 1:36-88.

on HP, Flynn JL. Latent tuberculosis: what the host "sees"? munol Res. 2011;50:202-12.

Lillebaek T, Dirksen A, Baess I, Strunge B, Omsen VO, Andersen AB. Molecular evidence of endogenous reactivation of Mycobacterium tuberculosis after 33 years of latent infection. J Infect Dis. 2002;185:401-4.

7. Lin PL, Flynn JL. Understanding latent tuberculosis: a moving target. J Immunol. 2010;185:15-22.
8. Nayak NC. Nature and evolution of pulmonary tuberculosis. J AIIMS. 1976;1:190-4.
9. Rhoades ER, Frank AA, Orme IM. Progression of chronic pulmonary tuberculosis in mice aerogenically infected with virulent Mycobacterium tuberculosis. Tubercle Lung Dis. 1997;78:57-66.
10. Saunders BM, Cooper AM. Restraining mycobacteria: role of granulomas in mycobacterial infections. Immunol Cell Biol. 2000;78:334-41.
11. Seal RM. The pathology of tuberculosis. Br J Hosp Med. 1971;5:783.
12. Vynnycky E, Fine PE. Lifetime risks, incubation period, and serial interval of tuberculosis. Am J Epidemiol. 2000;152:247-63.

CHAPTER 6
Clinical Presentation of Tuberculosis

INTRODUCTION

Exposure to *Mycobacterium tuberculosis* bacilli by an individual can be of no consequences to various manifestations with infection to disease. Clinical tuberculosis (TB) has been defined (Table 6.1) by the Center for Disease Control and American Thoracic Society based on the history of exposure to and/or infection with the bacilli into the following categories.

TABLE 6.1

\multicolumn{3}{l}{Clinical classification of tuberculosis based on exposure/infection/disease status}
Class	Type	Description
0	• No tuberculosis exposure • Not infected	• No history of exposure • Tuberculin skin test: negative
1	• Tuberculosis exposure • No evidence of infection	• History of exposure • Tuberculin skin test: negative
2	• Tuberculosis infection • No disease	• Positive tuberculin skin test • No clinical, bacteriologic, or radiographic evidence of tuberculosis

Continued

Clinical Presentation of Tuberculosis

Continued

Clinical classification of tuberculosis based on exposure/infection/disease status		
Class	Type	Description
3	• Tuberculosis • Clinically active	• Clinical, bacteriologic, or radiographic evidence of current disease. If the diagnosis is still pending, the person should be classified as a tuberculosis suspect (class 5). Person with past tuberculosis and who also currently has clinically active disease belongs to class 3. A person remains in class 3 until treatment for the current episode of disease is completed. This group is further defined by location of disease, bacteriologic status, chest radiograph finding, and tuberculin skin test
4	• Tuberculosis • Not clinically active	• History of episode(s) of tuberculosis Or • Abnormal but stable radiographic findings • Positive reaction to the tuberculin skin test • Negative bacteriologic studies And • No clinical or radiographic evidence of current disease
5	• Tuberculosis suspect	• Diagnosis pending • Tuberculosis disease should be ruled in or out within 3 months

Infection to disease is dependent on many risk factors and a complex interaction between the host and parasite besides a number of risk factors playing a major role. The risk of developing TB is shown in Table 6.2.

Clinical TB can present as:
- Congenital TB
- Primary TB
- Miliary TB
- Post-primary TB.

Clinic Consult Pulmonology: Tuberculosis

TABLE 6.2

Risk of developing tuberculosis	
Risk factor	*Estimated increased risk (compared with persons with no risk factors)*
Acquired immune deficiency syndrome	170
Human immunodeficiency virus infection	113
Kidney transplant	37
Silicosis	30
Chronic renal failure	10–25
Imunocompromised	4–16
Infection within past 2 years	15
Chest X-ray consistent with prior tuberculosis	2–14
Age <5 and >60	2–5
Diabetes mellitus	2–4

CONGENITAL TUBERCULOSIS

Congenital TB is a rare but fatal disease if untreated. It is defined as TB occurring in infants as a result of infection with *M. tuberculosis* during intrauterine life.

The criteria of making the diagnosis are as follows (Britzke's criteria):

- It should be bacteriologically proven
- The disease must be present within the first few days of life
- In cases presenting later in life, there must be a primary complex in the liver, or extrauterine infection must be excluded by separation from the mother at birth and segregation from any other possible source of infection.

As the above criteria is quite rigid, Cantwell et al. proposed a modification. Infant must have a proven tuberculous lesion and at least one of the following:

- Lesions in first week of life
- Primary hepatic complex or caseating hepatic granuloma

Clinical Presentation of Tuberculosis

- Tuberculosis infection of placenta or maternal genital tract
- Exclusion of postnatal transmission by thorough contact investigation.

Isolation of different patterns of restriction-fragment-length polymorphism in *M. tuberculosis* from the mother and the infant would exclude congenital transmission. Three modes of fetal infection have been proposed:

1. Hematogenous infection via the umbilical vein
2. Fetal aspiration of infected amniotic fluid
3. Fetal ingestion of infected amniotic fluid.

The form of disease has usually been miliary with multiple organ involvement. The lungs are almost always involved. Other frequently involved sites are liver, spleen, lymph node, the gastrointestinal tract, and kidneys. Nonspecific nature of symptoms during pregnancy and infancy makes early detection difficult. The affected infant is frequently born prematurely but signs of disease usually do not appear for several days or weeks. The most common signs are respiratory distress, fever, hepatosplenomegaly, poor feeding, lethargy and/or irritability, lymphadenopathy, and failure to thrive. Meningitis and jaundice are uncommon. In a small percentage of cases, otitis media, with or without mastoiditis, is the first sign of congenital TB. Papular or pustular skin lesions may be present. The Mantoux test is usually negative. Possible imaging findings are shown in Table 6.3. Positive smear and/or culture results

TABLE 6.3

Imaging findings in congenital tuberculosis	
Finding	Percentage of cases
Chest radiographic findings	
Normal	6.9%
Abnormal	–
Miliary tuberculosis	46.8%

Continued

Continued

Imaging findings in congenital tuberculosis	
Finding	*Percentage of cases*
Lobar pneumonia	11.8
Multiple pulmonary nodules	11.1%
Interstitial pneumonia	9.7%
Bronchopneumonia	9.7%
Mediastinal adenopathy	9.0%
Lung primary complex	1.4%
Pleuritis	0.7%
Abdominal imaging findings	**38**
Normal	10.5%
Abnormal multiple focal lesions in the liver and spleen	44.7%
Hepatosplenomegaly	34.2%
Liver primary complex	26.3%
Ascites	10.5%

can often be obtained from gastric washings open liver biopsy, lymph node biopsy, spinal fluid, ear discharge, endotracheal aspirate, or bone marrow aspirate.

PRIMARY TUBERCULOSIS

In the majority of cases, the primary infection is symptomless, and is passed off unnoticed. The only indication is a Mantoux conversion. A proportion will experience a short febrile illness. Only a small minority with severe infection or low host resistance will manifest with features of being unwell with anorexia, fretfulness, and failure to gain weight. The primary symptoms that develop due to an active TB infection are: tiredness or weakness, weight loss, fever, and night sweats. As lungs are the major organs to be affected, worsened symptoms, such as coughing, chest pain, hemoptysis, and shortness of breath, may also appear. Wheeze may be present because of compression of bronchial wall due to enlarged lymph nodes.

Pneumonia/Collapse

Dense homogenous radiologic shadows may be present in children due to enlarged lymph nodes compressing the bronchus. These may either be segmental or lobar. The right middle lobe is most commonly affected, because it is surrounded by a chain of lymph nodes at its origin and gets compressed easily (*middle lobe syndrome*).

Erythema Nodosum

Erythema nodosum is an inflammatory disorder that is tender, and appears as red bumps under the skin. It appears most commonly on the shins, but may occur on other areas of the body like buttocks, calves, ankles, thighs, and arms. The lesions begin as flat, firm, hot, red, and painful lumps approximately an inch across. Within a few days, they may become purplish, and then fade to a brownish, flat patch over several weeks. Other symptoms may include fever, general ill feeling (malaise), joint aches, skin redness, inflammation, irritation, or swelling of the leg or other affected area. The red and inflamed skin symptoms may regress to a bruise-like appearance. It has a characteristic racial distribution occurring in 1–2% of British and 5–15% of Scandinavian patients. It is very unusual in Asians or Black population and rare in individuals below the age of 7.

Phlyctenular Conjunctivitis

Allergic reaction of the conjunctiva caused by endogenous bacterial toxins and characterized by bleb or nodule formation near the limbus. May occur only in the bulbar conjunctiva (phlyctenular conjunctivitis), or simultaneously in the cornea and conjunctiva (phlyctenular keratoconjunctivitis), and sometimes in the cornea alone (phlyctenular keratitis). Phlctennular ophthelmia is a general term of all. Unlike erythema nodosum, which occurs in the first weeks of infection, it occurs within the first year.

Common in children and young adolescents, particularly from poor socioeconomic background. A number of conditions other than TB can cause this.

The condition may be associated with slight pyrexia, photophobia, excessive lacrimation, and with noses running, probably from the increased passage of tears down the nasal duct.

It is a kind of delayed hypersensitivity to the microorganism protein.

Pleural Effusion

Pleural effusion is sometimes seen with primary TB in children under puberty. Such effusions are small and transient. Large effusions are common after puberty.

Other Manifestations

Broncholiths or bronchiectasis may rarely be seen. Radiologically, the characteristic features of primary pulmonary TB are a focus of parenchymal lesion with involvement of ipsilateral hilar lymph nodes. Paratracheal node involvement may be seen in a substantial number of cases.

MILIARY TUBERCULOSIS

It is a form of disseminated TB produced by acute dissemination of tubercle bacilli through the blood stream. The term miliary is derived from the pathologic appearance of diffuse discrete nodular shadows each about the size of a millet seed (1–2 mm), which are characteristic of the classical disease. This results from a massive hematogenous dissemination of tubercle bacilli which are more or less uniformly distributed in the lungs and other viscera. Cryptic forms are not at all uncommon, they are common in older people and contribute an important proportion of cases of miliary TB and sometimes are diagnosed only at postmortem.

Clinical Presentation of Tuberculosis

The incidence may vary from 0.3 to 13.3% overall, but it is more common in children (0.7–41.3%). Distribution in the body is variable, the lungs are almost always involved. There may not be any physical sign except fever. Crepitations may be heard in later stages.

Hepatosplenomegaly, lymphadenopathy, and neck rigidity may be present. Other nonspecific symptoms and signs may be anorexia, weight loss, night sweats, weakness/fatigue, cough with or without sputum, chest pain, hemoptysis (rare), altered sensorium, seizures, abdominal pain, diarrhea, urinary symptoms, pallor, cyanosis, icterus, lymphadenopathy, ascites, and neurological signs. Others include pyrexia of unknown origin, pneumothorax/pneumomediastinum, myelophthisic anemia, acute empyema, septic shock, thyrotoxicosis, renal failure, sudden cardiac death, mycotic aneurysm of aorta, valvular endocarditis, and as incidental diagnosis, etc. Choroidal tubercles are present in over 90% of children, if looked carefully. The lesions are usually less than one-fourth of the diameter of the optic disk. Cryptic miliary or disseminated TB is seen usually in the elderly (>60 years) where it is difficult to diagnose. It may present as acute respiratory distress syndrome. The syndrome may develop after treatment. Immune-complex nephritis has been reported.

Hematologic changes associated with miliary TB of the bone marrow include lymphopenia in the peripheral blood, monocytopenia, and absence of giant cells in the bone marrow granulomata, and decreased iron stores in about one-third of the patients. Chest X-ray may be normal because the lesions are too small to be seen. When abnormal shadows are seen, they are evenly distributed and may vary from faint shadows, 1–2 mm in diameter to large dense shadows up to 5–10 mm. The shadows are usually uniform in size. Evidence of primary complex may be present. Bilateral, small, and pleural effusions may occur. A reticular pattern is rarely seen due to lymphatic involvement and is called lymphangitis reticularis tuberculosa. The shadows start disappearing slowly following treatment, taking up to 3–4 months on average. The lesions may calcify.

POST-PRIMARY TUBERCULOSIS

Post-primary TB is the most important type of clinical TB, because it is much frequent, and smear-positive sputum is the main source of infection responsible for the propagation and persistence of the disease in the community. The infected individual usually remains asymptomatic and can be diagnosed only with a positive tuberculin test reaction. Tuberculosis is more common in particular socioeconomic situations such as crowded living conditions, recent immigrations from high prevalence countries (for developed countries where this is one of the important factors), substance abuse, close contacts like household contacts, prisons, institutional residences, slum dwellers, residents of shelter homes, etc.

Classically, the onset of symptoms occurs over weeks to months. General symptoms like tiredness, malaise, weight loss, anorexia, and weakness are very common and reported by majority of patients. Fever with night sweats is a classical symptom of TB and more common in patients with more advanced form of the disease. Prolonged undiagnosed fever (pyrexia of unknown origin) is one of the common presentations of TB. Fever is present in up to 60% of patients, which disappears rapidly within 1–2 weeks with therapy. Most important symptom related to respiratory system includes cough. Duration of more than 2 weeks is a TB suspect in many TB control programs. Diagnosis of TB will be in around 12–15% of cases. Sputum may be mucoid, purulent, or blood-stained. Hemoptysis is a classical symptom, and may vary from mere blood staining of the sputum to massive amount of bleeding.

Chest pain is common and may vary from a dull ache or tightness to pleuritic pain, but distinctly different from

Clinical Presentation of Tuberculosis

that due to lung cancer. Elderly patients (>65 years) with TB are more likely to present with nonspecific complaints and atypical radiographic appearance. They usually have lower body weight, less hemoptysis, and more nonspecific symptoms. Various cytokines are thought to be responsible for the clinical manifestations of TB. Fever is a part of the acute phase reaction to immune challenge and is complex coordinated autonomic, neuroendocrine, and behavioral response. Fever might be initiated by an endogenous substance secreted during inflammation (endogenous pyrogen) rather than due to direct effect of the mycobacteria. The pyrogenic cytokines include interleukin (IL)-1β, IL-6, tumor necrosis factor (TNF)-α, and interferon (IFN), of which IL-6 has least pyrogenic action. Though the mechanisms of weight loss are not well known, but cachectin and TNF are thought to be responsible, particularly, the latter which induces catabolic response. Pleuritis and pleural effusion are thought to be due to TNF-α and IFN-γ. Tuberculosis can also produce features like acute respiratory distress syndrome. Lipoarabinomannan, a component of mycobacterial cell wall acts in a similar fashion to that of lipopolysaccharide in Gram-negative sepsis to activate macrophages to release various cytokines in the causation of lung injury.

There may be no physical signs of TB even with relatively advanced disease. However, fever, anemia, and cachexia will be present. Advanced cases may show finger clubbing. The earliest chest sign is a post-tussive crepitation in the upper lobes or apices. With the advancement of the disease, fibrosis with cavity is the most common finding in post-primary TB. The findings are most often bilateral. There may be signs of consolidation also when the presentation is like pneumonia. Loss of lung volume in chronic cases is very common. Clinical findings of collapse are not the findings of TB except in very young individuals due to node compression. Bronchostenosis may produce collapse. Localized wheezes are heard due to associated chronic bronchitis or rarely, due to bronchostenosis. Associated findings of pleural disease in the form of pleural effusion or pleural thickening may also be present.

Fibrothorax may be present in more advanced and chronic cases. Empyema or bronchopleural fistula is other clinical finding. Post-tubercular bronchiectasis, usually in the upper lobes may be present. Examination of the respiratory system is very important and findings of a cavity with fibrosis in association with history will strongly point toward TB as the underlying cause particularly in countries with high prevalence of the disease. Poncet's disease is an entity described as a reactive arthritis due to tuberculous infection elsewhere. Otherwise known as "tuberculous rheumatism," and "tuberculous reactive arthritis." It is thought to occur due to a hypersensitive immune cell mediated response to the tuberculoprotein, resulting in an inflammatory reaction in the joint spaces. It links to the human leukocyte antigen (HLA)-DR3 and HLA-DR4 haplotypes. Poncet's arthritis is nondestructive and resolves completely following TB treatment.

The differential diagnosis of pulmonary TB includes pneumonia, bronchogenic carcinoma, lung abscess, bacterial bronchiectasis, and fungal infections, which can be differentiated by their specific clinical findings.

COMPLICATIONS OF TUBERCULOSIS

Complications of pulmonary tuberculosis can be either local or general.

Local

- Hemoptysis
- Tuberculous bronchiectasis
- Fungal ball or aspergilloma
- Tubercular endobronchitis and tracheitis
- Spontaneous pneumothorax
- Scar carcinoma
- Disseminated calcification of the lungs

Clinical Presentation of Tuberculosis

- Obstructive airway diseases
- Secondary pyogenic infections
- Empyema
- Hyperreactivity of the airways
- Chronic obstructive pulmonary disease
- Respiratory disability with pulmonary function impairment.

General

- Secondary amyloidosis
- Respiratory failure
- Pulmonary hypertension or cor pulmonale.

KEY MESSAGE

❑ Clinical features of tuberculosis may vary according to the type like congenital form or post-primary forms of tuberculosis. Constitutional and respiratory symptoms are the common symptoms. Cough for more that two weeks is a good indicator and used by RNTCP that defines the subject as a TB suspect. The person needs to be invstigated further like a chest skiagram or sputum examination for the presence of *M. tuberculosis*. Sometimes, symptoms may be very nonspecific.

SUGGESTED READINGS

1. Behera D. Tuberculosis. In: Textbook of pulmonarymedicine. Ist ed. Jaypee Brothers Medical Publishers (P) Ltd.: New Delhi; 1995. p. 233-86.
2. Behera D. Complications of pulmonary tuberculosis. In: Sharma SK, Mohan A, editors. Tuberculosis. 2nd ed. Jaypee Brothers Medical Publishers (P) Ltd.: New Delhi; 2009. p. 519-31.
3. Beitzke H. Uber die angeborene tuberkulose infection. Ergeb Ges Tuberk Forsch. 1935;7:1-30.
4. Cantwell M, Snider DE Jr, Cauthen GM, Onorato IM. Epidemiology of tuberculosis in the United States, 1985 through 1992. JAMA. 1994;272:535-9.

5. Cantwell MF, Shehab ZM, Costello AM, Sands L, Green WF, Ewing EP, et al. Brief report: congenital tuberculosis. N Engl J Med. 1994;330:1051-4.
6. Diagnostic standards and classification of tuberculosis in adults and children. Official statement of the American Thoracic Society, the Centers for Disease Control and Prevention and the Infectious Diseases Society of America, 1999. Am J Respir Crit Care Med. 2000;161:1376-95.
7. Gelfand DA, Dinarello CA, Wolff SM. Fever of unknown origin. In: Isselbacher KJ, Braunwald E, Wilsomn JD, Martin JB, Fauci AS, Kasper DL, editors. Harrison's principles of internal medicine. Mcgraw-Hill Inc.: New York; 1994. p. 84.
8. Hatzistamatiou Z, Kaleyias J, Ikonomidou U, Papathoma E, Prifti E, Kostalos C. Congenital tuberculous lymphadeninitisin a preterm infant in Greece. Acta Paediatr. 2003;92:392-4.
9. Kinsey HI. Phlyctenular conjunctivitis in relation to tuberculosis in Children. Can Med Assoc J. 1932;26:199-301.
10. Naouri B, Virkud V, Malecki J, Mateo J, Narita M, Ashkin D, et al. Congenital pulmonary tuberculosis associated with maternal cerebral tuberculosis--Florida, 2002. MMWR Morb Mortal Wkly Rep. 2005;54(10):249-50.
11. Sahn SA, Neff TA. Miliay tuberculosis. Am J Med. 1974;56:494-505.
12. Saper CB, Christopher DB. The neurological basis of fever. N Engl J Med. 1994;330:1880-6.
13. Sbarbaro JA. Tuberculosis. Med Clin North Am. 1980;64:417-31.
14. Schaaf HS, Collins A, Bekker A, Davies PD. Tuberculosis at extremes of age. Respirology. 2010;15:747-63.
15. Schwartz RA, Nervi SJ. Erythema nodosum: a sign of systemic disease. Am Fam Physician. 2007;75:695-700.
16. Seaton A, Seaton D, Leitch AG. Clinical features of tuberculosis. In: Ayvazian LF, editor. Crofton and Doughlas's Respiratory Diseases. 4th ed. Blackwell Scientific Publications: London; 1989. p. 395-422.
17. Sharma SK, Mohan A, Sharma A, Mitra DK. Miliary tuberculosis: new insights into an old disease. Lancet Infect Dis. 2005;5:415-30.
18. Stead WW, Dutt AK. Tuberculosis in elderly persons. Annu Rev Med. 1991;42:267-76.
19. Stead WW, Eichenholz A, Stauss H. Operative and pathological changes in 24 patients with syndrome of idiopathic pleurisy with effusion, presumably tuberculous. Am Rev Tuberc. 1955;71:473-502.
20. Wang JY, Hsue PR, Wang SK, Jan IS, Lee LN, Liaw YS, et al. Disseminated tuberculosis: a 10 years experience in a medical center. Medicine (Baltimore). 2007;86:39-46.

CHAPTER 7

Radiology of Tuberculosis

INTRODUCTION

Tuberculosis (TB) can mimic any form of other chest diseases. All components of the respiratory system like the lung parenchyma, mediastinal and hilar nodes, bronchial tree, the pleura, vessels, and even the chest wall can be involved. However, there are certain important clues that can direct towards tuberculosis. Although it is most often needed to have a bacteriological/microbiological confirmation for its diagnosis (which is possible only in about a half of the cases), in an appropriate clinical setting certain radiological findings can be highly suggestive of tuberculosis. Computed tomography (CT) scan can sometimes add to some of the hidden findings missed on simple plane radiography.

Radiologic features of TB can almost mimic to any other form of respiratory disease. However, some generalizations can be made. A normal chest X-ray almost always excludes post-primary TB except under two conditions: (i) when there is an observer error and a small radiologic lesion is often missed and (ii) localized post-primary endobronchial TB may produce positive sputum, but normal chest X-ray. There are certain characteristic appearances which strongly suggest TB (but not exclusively due to TB) and they are: opacities in the upper zones, patchy or nodular opacities, presence of one or more cavities, presence of calcification, bilateral opacities particularly in the upper zones, and persistent shadows for weeks. Post-primary TB most commonly involves the apical and posterior segments of the upper lobes and the superior segments of the lower lobes. Some of the typical post-primary TB as seen on radiology are depicted below. Certain radiologic appearances suggest activity: a cavity, unless there has been previous effective treatment (isoniazid cavities are usually inactive); soft shadows; and shadows which extend on serial X-rays.

Computed tomography (CT) appearances of pulmonary TB include nodular opacities, consolidation, and consolidation with associated loss of volume. The diabetics and immunocompromised subjects will have a nonsegmental distribution and multiple small cavitations within any given lesion. Unusual localizations are also possible. Furthermore, centrilobular lesions (nodules or branching linear structures 2–4 mm in diameter) are most common findings. Most of these lesions disappear within 5 months of treatment. Computed tomography can also differentiate between old fibrotic and recent activation of TB. Lesions in and around the small airways appear to be the most characteristic CT features of early active TB and may be a reliable criterion for disease activity.

Classically, post-primary pulmonary TB is located predominantly in the upper lobes. However, it is not uncommon to find TB in the lower lung fields. Lower lung field is defined as the area on the posteroanterior chest radiograph that extends below an imaginary horizontal line traced across the hilum including the parahilar region. Prevalence of lower lung field varies between 0.003 and 15.8% of all cases of pulmonary TB. The condition is more common in patients receiving corticosteroids, patients with diabetes mellitus, hepatic or renal disease, pregnancy, scoliosis, and

Radiology of Tuberculosis

kyphoscoliosis. Various possible radiological pictures of tuberculosis are shown in Figures 7.1 to 7.23.

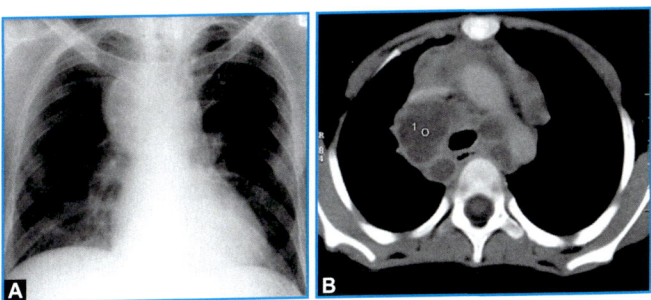

Figure 7.1 Tuberculous mediastinal lymphadenopathy. **A,** Right paratracheal lymphadenopathy. **B,** Contrast-enhanced computed tomography reveals low density center with peripheral rim enhancement of the node. Similar but smaller nodes are also seen in the posterior mediastinum.

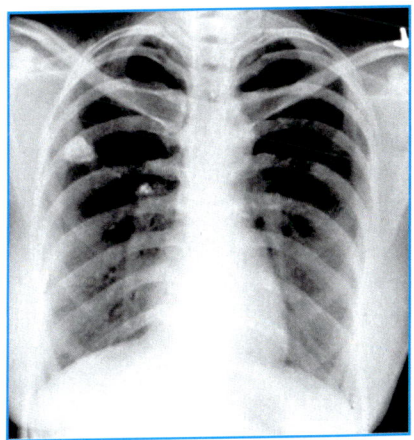

Figure 7.2 Primary complex. Calcified lesion in the right upper zone along with calcification of the right hilar node and of the intervening lymphatic channel.

Clinic Consult Pulmonology: Tuberculosis

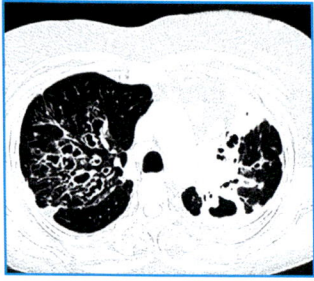

Figure 7.3 Diffuse varicose pattern of bronchiectasis on the right side. In addition, fibrocavitary changes on the left side.

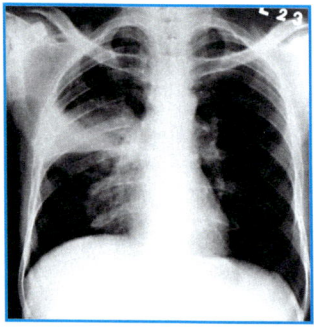

Figure 7.4 Primary tuberculosis in adult. Multilobar consolidation of the right lung affecting the upper and lower lobes without lymphadenopathy.

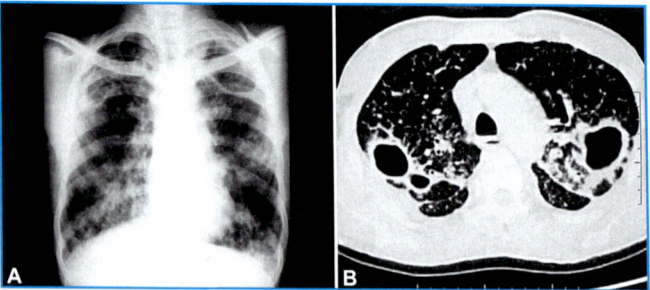

Figure 7.5 Post-primary tuberculosis. **A,** Cavitory lesions in both the upper lobes and multiple ill-defined nodular opacities in both the lung fields. **B,** High resolution computed tomography section in the region of the upper lobes shows bilateral thick walled cavities with surrounding consolidation.

Radiology of Tuberculosis

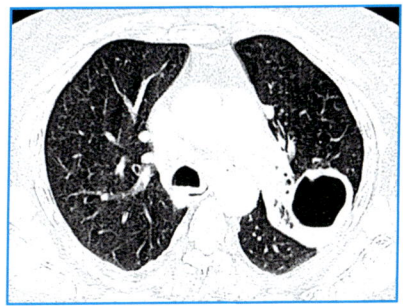

Figure 7.6 Well-defined smooth walled cavity in the left upper lobe. Minimal fluid level is also seen.

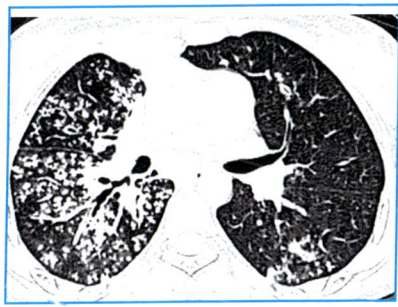

Figure 7.7 Diffusely distributed centrilobular nodules on the right side, indicative of endobronchial spread of infection. Few nodules are also seen on left side.

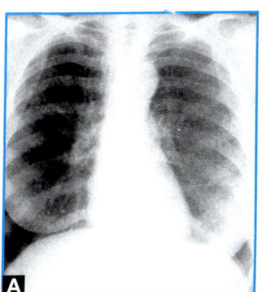 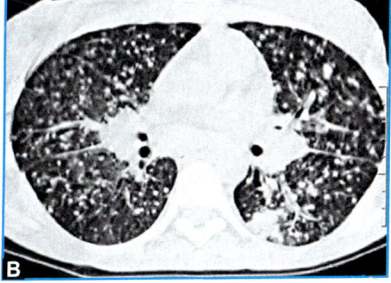

Figure 7.8 Miliary tuberculosis. **A,** Chest radiograph shows diffuse fine micronodular opacities in both lungs. **B,** High resolution computed tomography demonstrates peribronchiolar and perivascular nodules with air space consolidation in the superior segment of left lower lobe.

Clinic Consult Pulmonology: Tuberculosis

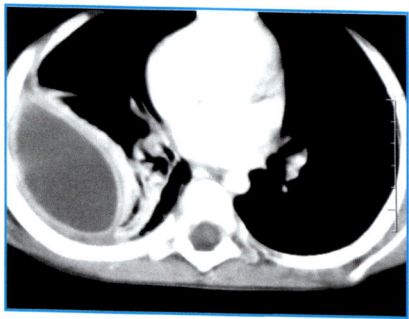

Figure 7.9 Empyema. Contrast-enhanced computed tomography chest depicting right pleural effusion with enhancing visceral and parietal pleura giving split-pleura sign.

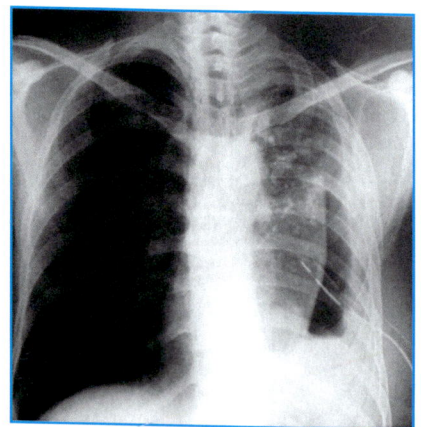

Figure 7.10 Bronchopleural fistula in a patient with nonresolving hydropneumothorax on intercostal tube drainage. Chest radiograph shows left pleural effusion with an air fluid level and partial atelectasis of the left lung.

Radiology of Tuberculosis

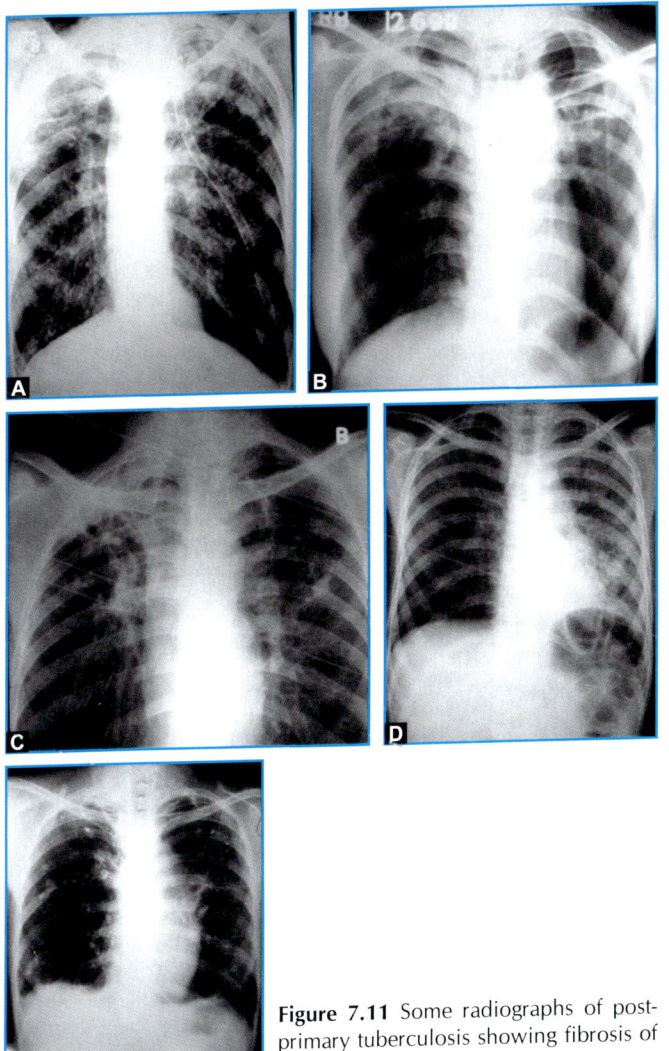

Figure 7.11 Some radiographs of post-primary tuberculosis showing fibrosis of lung parenchyma.

Clinic Consult Pulmonology: Tuberculosis

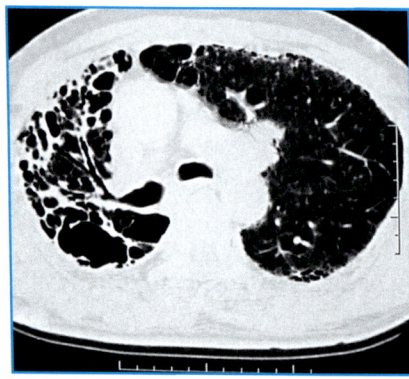

Figure 7.12 High resolution computed tomography shows traction bronchiectasis in the right upper lobe.

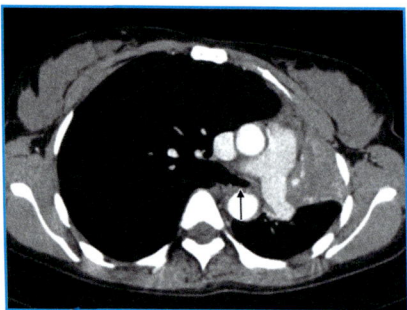

Figure 7.13 Axial contrast-enhanced computed tomography section (mediastinal window) showing circumferential thickening (arrow) of the wall of left upper lobe bronchus with distal collapse.

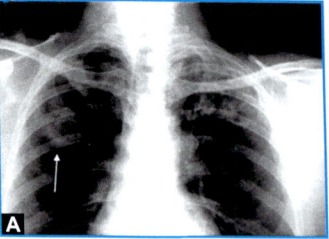 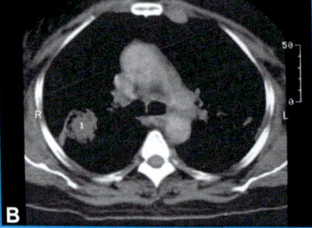

Figure 7.14 Mycetoma in a cavity. **A,** Cavity in the right upper lobe with a nodular lesion inside (arrow). **B,** Contrast-enhanced computed tomography of chest showing soft tissue (labelled as 1) filling the cavity with an air crescent anteriorly.

Radiology of Tuberculosis

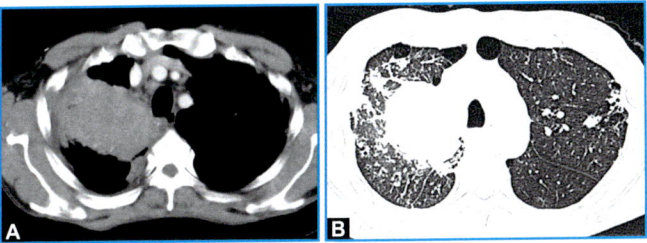

Figure 7.15 Scar carcinoma. **A,** Axial mediastinal window contrast-enhanced computed tomography section showing a large soft tissue mass in the left upper lobe suggestive of carcinoma. **B,** A lung window showing fibrotic changes due to old healed tubercular infection in bilateral upper lobes. Paraseptal emphysematous changes are also seen bilaterally.

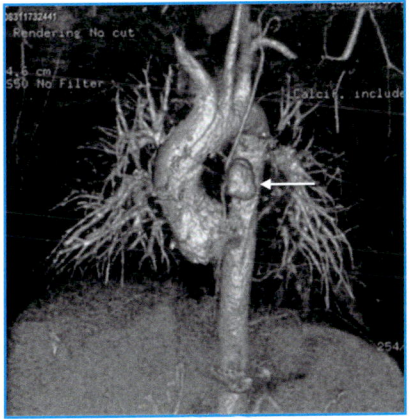

Figure 7.16 Reconstructed volume rendered image of computed tomography angiography showing pseudo-aneurysm (arrow) arising from left internal mammary artery (LIMA) which was formed due to pocket of tubercular empyema located encasing the LIMA in the anterior aspect. *(For color version, see Plate 7)*

Clinic Consult Pulmonology: Tuberculosis

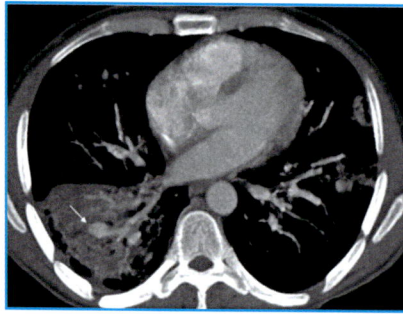

Figure 7.17 Axial maximum intensity projection image of a 45-year old man with massive hemoptysis showing a pseudoaneurysm (arrow) from the branch of right pulmonary artery.

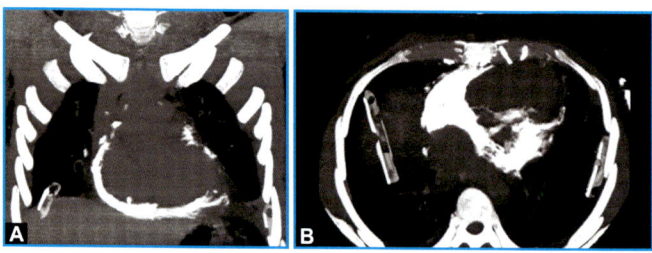

Figure 7.18 A, Coronal and **B,** axial thick maximum intensity projection images showing dense and thick pericardial calcification in a patient with past history of tuberculosis.

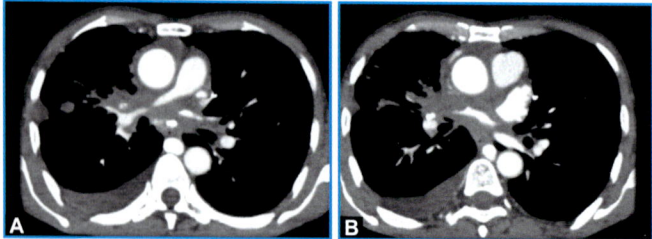

Figure 7.19 Axial mediastinal window sections showing sheet like soft tissue within the mediastinum encasing the major vessels. In addition, calcified lymph nodes are also seen. Pleural effusion is also seen on the right side.

Radiology of Tuberculosis

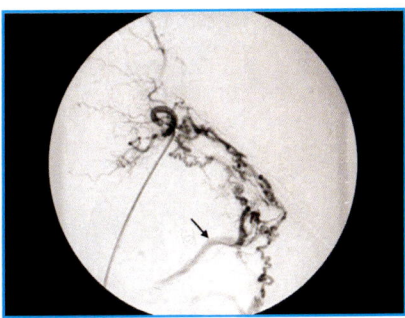

Figure 7.20 Selective left bronchial angiogram showing bronchopulmonary fistula evidenced by early opacification of the pulmonary venous branches (arrow).

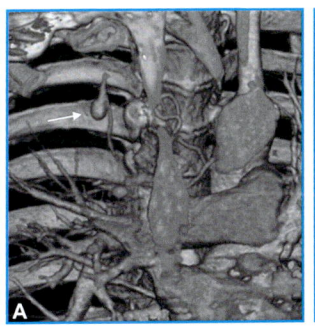
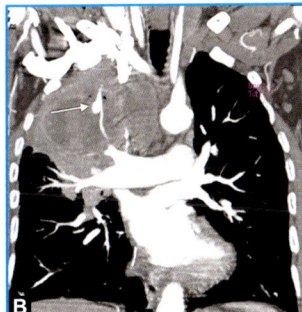
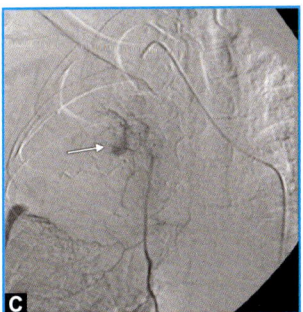

Figure 7.21 A, Volume rendering and **B,** coronal maximum intensity projection images showing a pseudoaneurysm in right upper lobe (arrows in A and B) arising from internal mammary artery (IMA). Surrounding consolidation is also seen. **C,** Selective right IMA run showing the pseudoaneurysm (arrow). *(For color version, see Plate 7)*

Clinic Consult Pulmonology: Tuberculosis

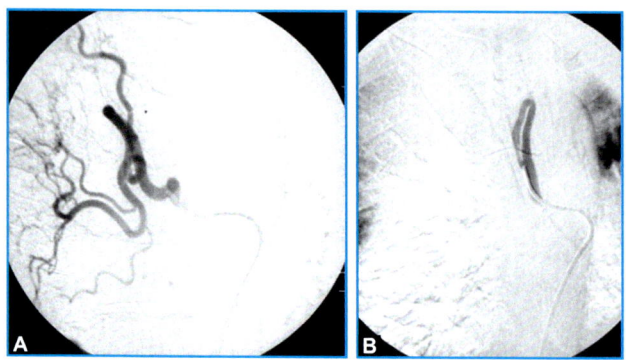

Figure 7.22 Selective right bronchial angiogram shows enlarged and tortuous right bronchial artery. Postembolization angiography run of right bronchial artery.

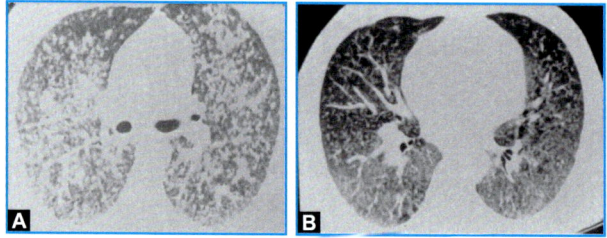

Figure 7.23 On the left hand side the nodules are centri-nodular and diffuse (tuberculosis) vs perilymphatic and peribronchovascular distribution of nodules in sarcoidosis (right hand side).

The National Tuberculosis Association of the USA has classified the radiologic extent TB in to three types (Table 7.1).

TABLE 7.1

Radiological classification of extent of pulmonary tuberculosis	
Extent	*Radiological findings*
Minimal	The lesions are slight to moderate in density, but no demonstrable cavities. The extent of involvement may be a small part of one or both lungs, but the total extent, regardless of distribution, should not exceed the volume of lung on one side, which is present above the second chondrosternal junction, and the spine of the 4th or the body of the 5th thoracic vertebra
Moderately advanced	This may be present in one or both lungs, but the total extent should not exceed the following limits: disseminated lesions of slight to moderate density which may extend throughout the total volume of one lung, or the equivalent of both lungs; dense and confluent lesions which are limited in extent to one-third the volume of one lung; and total diameter of cavitation, if present, should be less than 4 cm
Far advanced	Lesions more extensive than moderately advanced

KEY MESSAGE

❑ Although radiological picture of tuberculosis may mimic other lung diseases, there may be certain characeristic features that may suggest pulmonary tuberculosis. All components of the lungs may be involved like the mediastinal nodes, parenchyma, and the airways. Computed tomographic features are quite characteristics of the disease that may distinguish them from other non-tubercular lung diseases.

SUGGESTED READINGS

1. Burrill F, Williams CJ, Bain G, Conder G, Hine AL, Misra RR. Tuberculosis: a radiologic review. Radiographics. 2007;27:1255-73.
2. Choyke PL, Sostman HD, Curtis AM, Ravin CE, Chen JT, Godwin JD, et al. Adult-onset pulmonary tuberculosis. Radiology. 1983;148:357-62.
3. Forbes TL, Harris JR, Nie RG, Lawlor DK. Tuberculous aneurysm of the supraceliac aorta--a case report. Vasc Endovasc Surg. 2004;38:93-7.
4. Geng E, Kreiswirth B, Burzynski J, Schluger NW. Clinical and radiographic correlates of primary and reactivation tuberculosis: a molecular epidemiology study. JAMA. 2005;293:2740-5.
5. Gyselen A, Uydebroeck M, Weyler J. Epidemiologie. In: Demedts M, Gyselen A, Van den Brande P, editors. Tuberculosis. Een blijvende uitdaging. Leuven-Apeldoorn: Garant; 1992. p. 17-30.
6. Hadlock FP, Park SK, Awe RJ, Rivera M. Unusual radiographic findings in adult pulmonary tuberculosis. Am J Roentgenol. 1980;134:1015-8.
7. Haponik EF, Britt EJ, Smith PL, Bleecker ER. Computed chest tomography in the evaluation of hemoptysis: impact on diagnosis and treatment. Chest. 1987;91:80-5.
8. Harkirat S, Anand SS, Indrajit IK, Dash AK. Pictorial essay: PET/CT in tuberculosis. Indian J Radiol Imaging. 2009;18:141-7.
9. Im JG, Itoh H, Shim YS, Lee JH, Ahn J, Han MC, et al. Pulmonary tuberculosis: CT finding—early active disease and sequential change with antituberculous therapy. Radiology. 1993;186:653-60.
10. Im JG, Webb WR, Han MC, Park JH. Apical opacity associated with pulmonary tuberculosis: high-resolution CT findings. Radiology. 1991;178:727-31.
11. Jeong YJ, Lee KS. Pulmonary tuberculosis: Up-to-date imaging and management. Am J Roentgenol. 2008;191:834-44.
12. Kim HY, Song KS, Goo JM, Lee JS, Lee KS, Lim TH. Thoracic sequelae and complications of tuberculosis. Radiographics. 2001;21:839-60.
13. Kwong JS, Carignan S, Kang EY, Müller NL, FitzGerald JM. Miliary tuberculosis: diagnostic accuracy of chest radiography. Chest. 1996;110:339-42.
14. Lamont AC, Cremin BJ, Pelteret RM. Radiologic patterns of pulmonary tuberculosis in the paediatric age group. Paediatr Radiol. 1986;16:2-7.

15. Lee KS, Song KS, Lim TH, Kim PN, Kim IY, Lee BH. Adult-onset pulmonary tuberculosis: findings on chest radiographs and CT scans. Am J Roentgenol. 1993;160:753-8.
16. Leung AN, Muller NL, Pineda PR, FitzGerald JM. Primary tuberculosis in childhood: radiographic manifestations. Radiology. 1992;182:87-91.
17. Leung AN. Pulmonary tuberculosis: the essentials. Radiology. 1999;210:307-22.
18. Palmer PE. Pulmonary tuberculosis: usual and unusual radiographic presentations. Semin Roentgenol. 1979;14:204-42.
19. Ponnuswamy I, Sankaravadivelu ST, Maduraimuthu P, Natarajan K, Sathyanathan BP, Sadras S. 64-detector row CT evaluation of bronchial and non-bronchial systemic arteries in life-threatening hemoptysis. Br J Radiol. 2012;85:666-72.
20. Santelli ED, Katz DS, Goldschmidt AM, Thomas HA. Embolization of multiple Rasmussen aneurysms as a treatment of hemoptysis. Radiology. 1994;193:396-8.
21. Woodring JH, Vandiviere HM, Fried AM, Dillon ML, Williams TD, Melvin IG. Update: radiographic features of pulmonary tuberculosis. Am J Roentgenol. 1986;146:497-506.

Acknowledgment

The author would like to thank Dr Mandeep Garg, Associate Professor, Department of Radiodiagnosis, Postgraduate Institute of Medical education and Research, Chandigarh for granting permission to use radiograph images for this chapter.

CHAPTER 8
Laboratory Diagnosis of Tuberculosis

INTRODUCTION

Early and accurate diagnosis is critical to start treatment early to break the chain of transmission. The best practices for tuberculosis (TB) care are incorporated in the International Standards of TB Care (ISTC), which was first published in 2006. The Indian standards of TB care also mentions six components for diagnosis.

Standard 1: Testing and Screening for Pulmonary Tuberculosis

- Testing: any person with symptoms and signs suggestive of TB, including cough more than 2 weeks, fever more than 2 weeks, significant weight loss, hemoptysis, and any abnormality in chest radiograph must be evaluated for TB. Children with persistent fever and/or cough more than 2 weeks, loss of weight/no weight gain, and/or contact with pulmonary TB cases must be evaluated for TB
- Screening: people living with human immunodeficiency virus, malnourished, diabetics, cancer patients, patients on immunosuppressant, or maintenance steroid therapy should be regularly screened for signs and symptoms suggestive of TB. Enhanced case finding should be undertaken in high risk populations, such as healthcare workers, prisoners, slum dwellers, and certain occupational groups such as miners.

Laboratory Diagnosis of Tuberculosis

Standard 2: Diagnostic Technology

- Microbiological confirmation on sputum: all patients (adults, adolescents, and children who are capable of producing sputum) with presumptive pulmonary TB should undergo quality-assured sputum test for rapid diagnosis of TB [with at least two samples, including one early morning sample for sputum smear for acid-fast bacillus (AFB)] for microbiological confirmation
- Chest X-ray as screening tool: where available, chest X-ray should be used as a screening tool to increase the sensitivity of the diagnostic algorithm
- Serological tests: serological tests are banned and not recommended for diagnosing TB
- Tuberculin skin test (TST) and interferon-γ release assay (IGRA): TST and IGRA are not recommended for the diagnosis of active TB. Standardized TST may be used as a complimentary test in children
- Cartridge-based nucleic-acid amplification test (CB-NAAT): it is the preferred first diagnostic test in children and people living with human immunodeficiency virus
- Validation of newer diagnostic tests: effective mechanism should be developed to validate newer diagnostic tests. Children with persistent fever and/or cough more than 2 weeks, loss of weight/no weight gain, and/or contact with pulmonary TB cases must be evaluated for TB.

Standard 3: Testing for Extrapulmonary Tuberculosis

For all patients (adults, adolescents, and children) with presumptive extrapulmonary TB, appropriate specimens from the presumed sites of involvement must be obtained for microscopy/culture and drug sensitivity testing (DST)/CB-NAAT/molecular test/histopathological examination.

Standard 4: Diagnosis of Human Immunodeficiency Virus Coinfection in Tuberculosis Patients and Drug-resistant Tuberculosis

All diagnosed TB patients should be offered HIV counseling and testing. Prompt and appropriate evaluation should be undertaken for patients with presumptive MDR-TB or rifampicin (R) resistance in TB patients who have failed treatment with first line drugs, pediatric nonresponders, TB patients who are contacts of MDR-TB (or R resistance), TB patients who are found positive on any follow-up sputum smear examination during treatment with first line drugs, diagnosed TB patients with prior history of anti-TB treatment, TB patients with HIV co-infection, and all presumptive TB cases among PLHIV. All such patients must be tested for drug resistance with available technology, a rapid molecular DST (as the first choice) or liquid/solid culture-DST (at least for R and if possible for isoniazid (H); ofloxacin (O) and kanamycin (K), if R-resistant/MDR). Wherever available, DST should be offered to all diagnosed tuberculosis patients prior to start of treatment. On detection of rifampicin resistance alone or along with isoniazid resistance, patient must be offered sputum test for second line DST using RNTCP approved phenotypic or genotypic methods, wherever available.

Standard 5: Probable Tuberculosis

Presumptive TB patients without microbiological confirmation (smear microscopy, culture, and molecular diagnosis), but with strong clinical and other evidence (e.g., X-ray, fine needle aspiration cytology, histopathology) may be diagnosed as "probable TB" and should be treated. For patients with presumptive TB found to be negative on rapid molecular test, an attempt should be made to obtain culture on an appropriate specimen.

Standard 6: Pediatric Tuberculosis

- Diagnosis of pediatric TB patients: in all children with presumptive intrathoracic TB, microbiological confirmation should be sought through examination of respiratory specimens (e.g., sputum by expectoration, gastric aspirate, gastric lavage, induced sputum, bronchoalveolar lavage, or other appropriate specimens) with an quality assured diagnostic test, preferably CB-NAAT, smear microscopy, or culture
- Diagnosis of probable pediatric TB patients
- Diagnosis of extrapulmonary pediatric TB patients.

DIAGNOSIS OF ACTIVE TUBERCULOSIS

Active TB, ideally, should be microbiologically confirmed. There are three methods that are recommended for microbiological confirmation of active TB disease:
1. Smear microscopy
2. Cultures
3. Nucleic acid amplification tests.

Smear Microscopy

Smear microscopy is a rapid, inexpensive, and widely available technology. While sensitivity is modest (50–70%), specificity is very high (>98%). Three methods are usually adopted: Ziehl-Neelsen staining, conventional, and light-emitting diode (LED)-based fluorescent microscopy. Mycobacteria are "acid-fast bacilli" because of their lipid-rich cell walls, which are relatively impermeable to various basic dyes unless the dyes are combined with phenol. Once stained, the cells resist decolorization with acidified organic solvents and are, therefore, called "acid-fast" (other bacteria, which also contain mycolic acids, such as *Nocardia*, can also exhibit this feature).

Clinic Consult Pulmonology: Tuberculosis

Mycobacteria are extremely difficult to stain by Gram-stain because of the high lipid content of the cell wall. The phenolic compound carbol fuchsin is used as the primary stain because it is lipid soluble and penetrates the waxy cell wall. Staining by carbol fuchsin is further enhanced by steam heating the preparation to melt the wax and allowing the stain to move into the cell. Acid is used to decolorize nonacid-fast cells; acid-fast cells resist this decolorization. The ability of the bacteria to resist decolorization with acid confers acid-fastness to the bacterium. Following decolorization, the smear is counterstained with malachite green or methylene blue which stains the background material, providing a contrast colour against which the red AFB can be seen. Acid alcohol can also be used as decolorizing solution, resistant organisms are referred to as acid fast bacilli (AFB).

To make the staining, a thin smear of the material should be prepared for study and then heat fixed by passing the slide 3–4 times through the flame of a Bunsen burner. It should not be overheated. Then the slide is placed on the staining rack and carbol fuschin is poured over the smear and heated gently to the underside of the slide by passing a flame under the rack until fumes appear (without boiling!). It should not be overheated and then allowed to stand for 5 minutes. Then the smears is rinsed with water until no color appears in the effluent. Then 20% sulphuric acid is poured after one minute and one should keep on repeating this step until the slide appears light pink in color (15–20 sec). The slide is then washed well with clean water. The smear is covered with methylene blue or malachite green stain for 1–2 minutes. The stain is washed off with clean water. The back of the slide is wiped off, cleaned, and then it is placed in a draining rack for the smear to air-dry (not to be blot dried). The smear is then examined microscopically, using the 100x oil immersion objective.

The acid fast bacilli appear as red, straight or slightly curved rods, occurring singly or in small groups. They may

Laboratory Diagnosis of Tuberculosis

also appear beaded against a green (malachite green) or blue (methylene blue) background (Figure 8.1).

acid fast organisms are:

1. *Mycobacterium spp.*: Acid fast
2. Cyst of cryptosporidium: Acid fast
3. Cyst of isospora:
4. Acid fast *Nocardia spp.*: Partial acid fast
5. *Rhodococcus spp.*: Partial acid fast
6. *Legionella micdadei*: Partially acid fast in tissue.

One needs presence of at least 10,000 mycobacteria/mL of sputum to get positivity. The sensitivity is reduced (over all ~59%) compared to culture. The sensitivity comes down to 25–40% in HIV cases due to lack of cavity and paucibacillary nature of HIV-TB. It will take two days to get the result. Based on several World Health Organization (WHO) policies, at least two sputum samples should be stained with a fluorescence stain and read by a well-trained microscopist using LED microscopy (Figure 8.2), in a laboratory that is engaged in an ongoing external quality assurance (EQA) program. Light-emitting diode microscopy is WHO-endorsed and already in use in several medical colleges in India in high burden settings. Recent research from India has clearly shown its impact

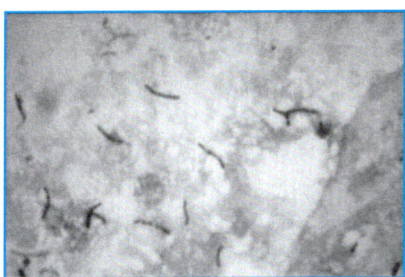

Figure 8.1 Acid-fast bacilli. Note red colored straight or slightly curved acid-fast bacilli. *(For color version, see Plate 8)*

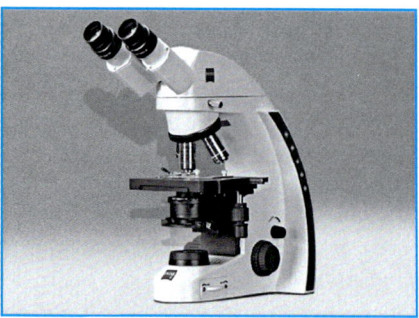

Figure 8.2 Light-emitting diode microscope.

in terms of increased sensitivity and case detection. It gives about 10% more yield. Thus, where possible, traditional Ziehl-Neelsen microscopy should be upgraded to LED fluorescence microscopy.

Cultures

Solid Culture

Culture of sputum provides definitive diagnosis of TB and establishes the viability and identity of organisms. Compared to other bacteria, which typically reproduce within minutes, *M. tuberculosis* proliferates extremely slowly (generation time 18–24 h). Growth requirements are such that it will not grow on primary isolation on simple chemically defined media. The only media that allow abundant growth of *M. tuberculosis* are egg-enriched media with glycerol and asparagine (viz., Löwenstein–Jensen) or agar based media supplemented with bovine albumin (viz., Middlebrook, 7H10 or 7H11). Culture increases the number of TB cases found, often by 30–50% and detects cases which are smear-negative.

Since culture techniques detect fewer bacilli, the efficiency of diagnosing cases of failure at end of treatment can be improved considerably. Cultures also provide sufficient material for drug susceptibility and identification tests. However, culture methods are expensive and require considerable expertise. Typical colonies of *M. tuberculosis* are rough, crumbly, waxy, nonpigmented (buff colored), and slow-growers, i.e., only appearing two to three weeks after inoculation. The growth time is between 6–8 weeks Figure 8.3.

This is no more used for primary use by the program, but useful for monthly follow-up of multidrug-resistant (MDR)-TB patients on treatment.

Liquid Culture

Liquid culture is the gold standard for active TB diagnosis. Commercial systems like BACTEC MGIT® 960 and BacT/ALERT 3D are WHO-endorsed and can provide results within 10–14 days, and mycobacteria growth indicator tube (MGIT) (Fig. 8.4) can provide phenotypic DST results for first line and select second line drugs. Mycobacteria growth indicator tube is intended for the detection and recovery of mycobacteria. The MGIT tube contains 7 mL of modified Middlebrook 7H9 broth base. The complete medium, with Dubos oleic albumin complex enrichment and PANTA (polymyxin B,

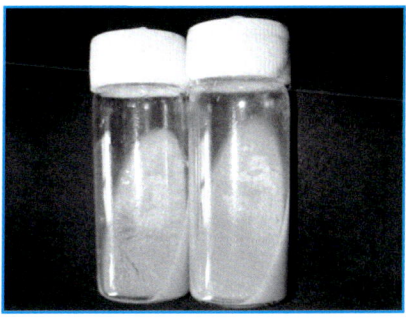

Figure 8.3 Note the growth of *Mycobacterium tuberculosis* in a Lowenstein Jensen media. *(For color version, see Plate 8)*

Clinic Consult Pulmonology: Tuberculosis

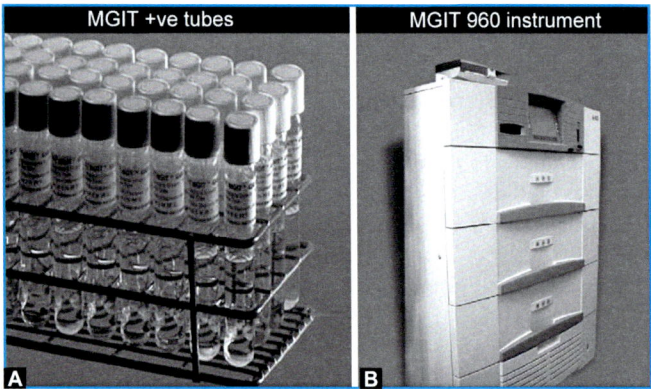

MGIT, mycobacteria growth indicator tube.

Figure 8.4 Mycobacterial growth indicator tube. *(For color version, see Plate 9)*

amphotericin B, nalidixic acid, trimethoprim, and azlocillin) antibiotic mixture, is one of the most commonly used liquid media for the cultivation of mycobacteria. All types of clinical specimens, pulmonary as well as extrapulmonary (except blood and urine) can be processed for primary isolation in the MGIT tube using conventional methods. After processed specimen is inoculated, MGIT tube must be continuously monitored. The fluorescent compound is sensitive to the presence of oxygen dissolved in the broth. Initially, the large amount of dissolved oxygen quenches emissions from the compound and little fluorescence can be detected. Later, actively respiring microorganisms consume the oxygen and allow the fluorescence to be detected. Reliability of second line DST is limited and, therefore, results should be carefully correlated with history of TB drugs taken in the past. Liquid culture also help in paucibacillary TB cases (extrapulmonary TB, smear-negative TB, and childhood TB). More sensitive and can be positive even when bacterial load is low (10–100 bacilli/mL).

Both manual and fully automated versions are available. Rapid detection (4–21 days) and DST (15–28 days) is possible. The main disadvantage is that one needs a biosafety level 3, which is expensive. Continuous power supply and air conditioning required. Chances of contamination is slightly higher, ~10%. Requirement of highly skilled man power.

Rapid Speciation of Positive Cultures

After the growth of the mycobacteria, species identification is required to differentiate it from the nontuberculous mycobacteria (NTM). Increased yield of NTMs with liquid cultures necessitates prompt identification of mycobacterial growth as TB versus NTM. Immunochromatographic tests by rapid strip test that detects a TB-specific antigen (MPB 64) from culture will be helpful. Bacterial growth derived from solid or liquid culture can be used. Typical is the Capilia test (Fig. 8.5). There will be a control band and a test band. If it is present then *M. tuberculosis* complex; if absent, not *M. tuberculosis* complex.

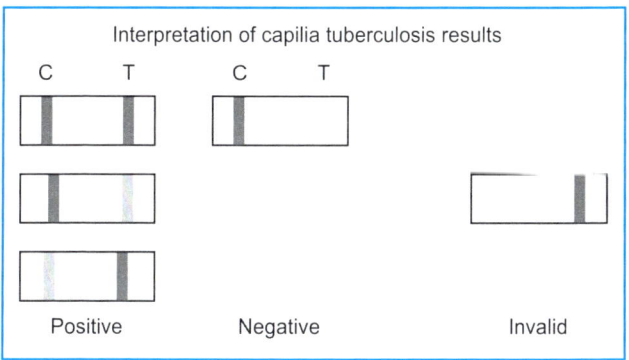

Figure 8.5 Capilia tuberculosis test to differentiate between species. *(For color version, see Plate 9)*

Nucleic acid Amplification Tests

Integrated Automated Nucleic Acid Amplification Test-GeneXpert

In 2010, the WHO endorsed a new, rapid, automated, 2-hour molecular test called Xpert MTB/RIF based on the GeneXpert technology for the detection of anthrax. The Xpert MTB/RIF detects DNA sequences specific for *M. tuberculosis* and rifampicin resistance by polymerase chain reaction. It is based on the Cepheid GeneXpert system, a platform for rapid and simple-to-use NAATs. It purifies and concentrates *M. tuberculosis* bacilli from sputum samples, isolates genomic material from the captured bacteria by sonication, and subsequently amplifies the genomic DNA by polymerase chain reaction (PCR). The process identifies all the clinically relevant rifampicin resistance inducing mutations in the RNA polymerase beta (rpoB) gene in the *M. tuberculosis* genome in a real time format using fluorescent probes called molecular beacons. Results are obtained from unprocessed sputum samples in 90 minutes, with minimal biohazard and very little technical training required to operate. This test was developed as an on-demand near patient technology which could be performed even in a doctor's office if necessary. There is onboard sample preparation with fully-automated reverse transcription-PCR amplification and detection. It is a Cartridge-based system that incorporates microfluidics technology and fully automated nucleic acid analysis. Machines with 1, 4, 16, and 48 modules are available, permitting multiple assays to be run concurrently and independently. It is specific for *M. tuberculosis* and the sensitivity is similar to culture. It detects rifampicin resistance via rpoB gene. The assay procedures are shown in Figure 8.6. The detection is based on the principle given in Figures 8.7 and 8.8.

Laboratory Diagnosis of Tuberculosis

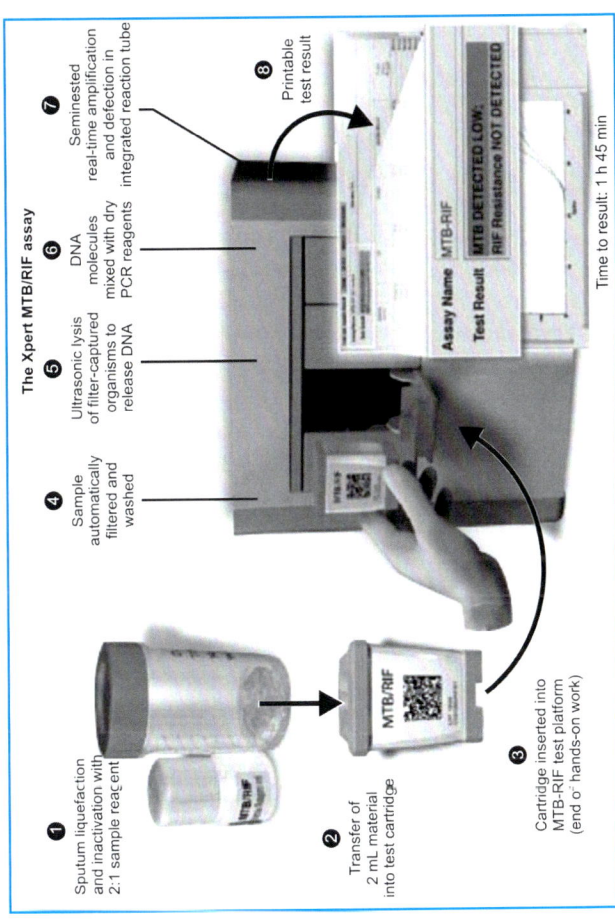

Figure 8.6 Gene'Xpert testing. *(For color version, see Plate 10)*

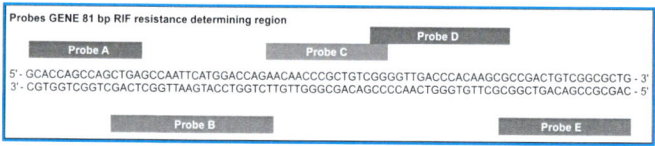

Figure 8.7: Gene probe for rifampicin resistance. *(For color version, see Plate 11)*

Although it detects the rifampicin resistance, it is almost similar to MDR as the key determinant for treatment failure is rifampicin resistance, detection of rifampicin resistance is taken as a proxy for MDR-TB. Almost all rifampicin-resistant isolates have mutation in the 81bp hotspot region *rpoB* (codon 507-533). Mutations are found in the rifampicin resistant determining region in 90–95% of resistant isolates. Major advantages in workflow as it is fully automated with 1-step external sample preparation. Time-to-result is one and half hour (walk away test). Up to 16 tests/module/run can be done. No biosafety cabinet required and being a closed system, there is no contamination risk.

A Cochrane review has shown that the Xpert MTB/RIF test has 88% sensitivity and 98% specificity when compared to culture. Even in smear-negative, culture-proven TB cases, Xpert has a sensitivity of about 68%. Xpert MTB/RIF can detect rifampicin resistance with a sensitivity of 95% and specificity of 98%. There are a number of disadvantages like the shelf life of the cartridges is only 18 months; very stable electricity supply is required; the instrument needs to be recalibrated annually; the cost of the test; and the temperature ceiling is critical. The main advantages of the test are for diagnosis and reliability when compared to sputum microscopy and the speed of getting the result when compared with culture. For diagnosis of TB, although sputum microscopy is both quick and cheap,

Laboratory Diagnosis of Tuberculosis

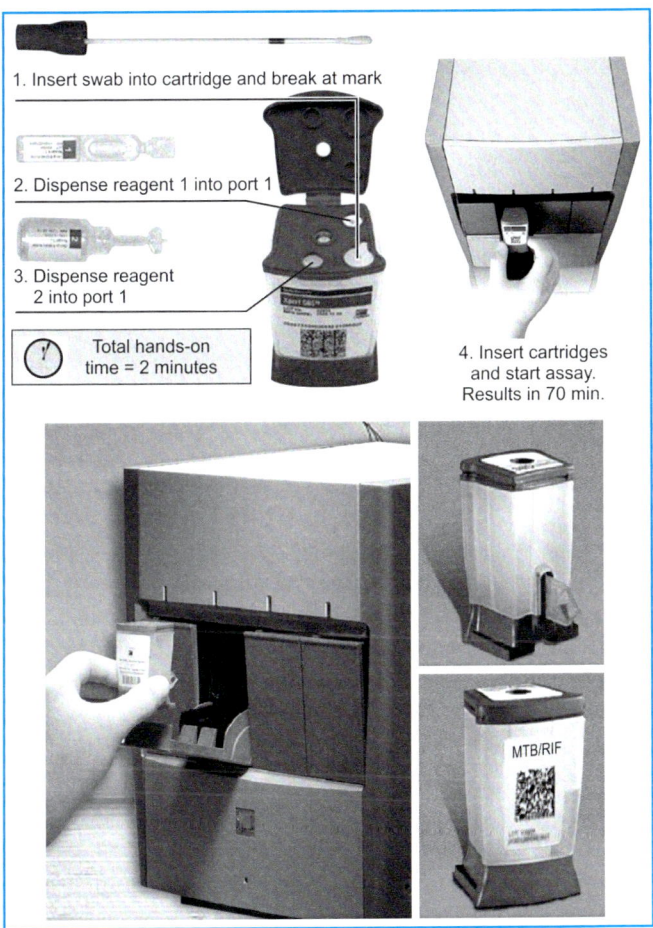

Figure 8.8 Steps up of Gene X pert test for detection of TB and Rif-resistance.

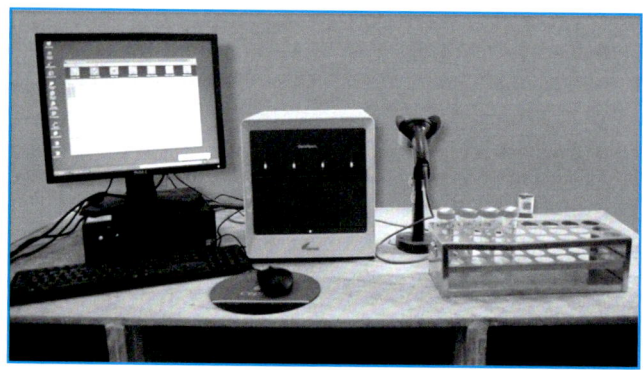

Figure 8.9 Cartridge-based nucleic acid amplification test laboratory of Revised National Tuberculosis Control Program of India.

it is often unreliable. It is particularly unreliable when people are HIV positive. Although culture gives a definitive diagnosis, to get the result usually takes weeks rather than the hours of the Xpert test. The main advantage in respect of identifying rifampicin resistance is, again, the matter of speed (Fig. 8.9). Normally, to get any drug resistance result takes weeks rather than hours. Data from many countries, including India, clearly show substantially better performance of the Xpert MTB/RIF test over conventional smear microscopy. Newer data also suggest that Xpert MTB/RIF has value for extrapulmonary TB, especially TB lymphadenitis and TB meningitis.

The 2013 recommendation of WHO for the use of Gene X'pert in the diagnosis of Pulmonary and extra-pulmonary tuberculosis is shown in Table 8.1.

Line Probe Assays

Line probe assays are designed to identify *M. tuberculosis* complex and simultaneously detect mutations associated

Laboratory Diagnosis of Tuberculosis

TABLE 8.1

Updated World Health Organization recommendations (October 2013)	
For diagnosis of pulmonary TB and rifampicin resistance	*For diagnosis of extrapulmonary TB and rifampicin resistance*

• Strong recommendation:
  • Xpert MTB/RIF should be used as the initial diagnostic test in adults and children presumed to have MDR-TB or HIV-associated TB
• Conditional recommendation (recognizing major resource implications):
  • Xpert MTB/RIF may be used as the initial diagnostic test in adults and children presumed to have TB
  • Xpert MTB/RIF may be used as a follow-on test to microscopy in adults presumed to have TB but not at risk of MDR-TB or HIV-associated TB, especially in further testing of smear-negative specimens
	• Strong recommendation:
	  • Xpert MTB/RIF should be used as the initial diagnostic test in testing cerebrospinal fluid specimens from patients presumed to have TB meningitis
	• Conditional recommendation:
	  • Xpert MTB/RIF may be used as a replacement test for usual practice (including conventional microscopy, culture, and/or histopathology) for testing of specific nonrespiratory specimens (lymph nodes and other tissues) from patients presumed to have extrapulmonary TB

TB, tuberculosis; MDR-TB, multidrug-resistant tuberculosis; HIV, human immunodeficiency virus.

with drug resistance. They are a family of novel DNA strip-based tests that use PCR and reverse hybridization methods for the rapid detection of mutations associated with drug resistance. Line probe assay has high sensitivity and specificity when culture isolates are used. The majority of studies had sensitivity of 95% or greater, and nearly all were

100% specific. There are two commercial assays available, namely, genotype MTBDRplus and INNO-LipA Rif. TB. The test is validated for use directly from smear-positive sputum (MTBDRplus) or from TB cultures. They can either be manual or automated systems. The TwinCubator is 10/run and the GT Blot is 48/run. It detects *rpoB* for rifampicin resistance (Inno-LiPA) and *rpoB* for rifampicin, and *katG* and *inhA* for isoniazid resistance by (MTBDRplus). Use of line probe assays is possible on smear-positive samples only. Line probe assays do not replace conventional culture + DST. Commercial assays recommend lab infrastructure, procedures and biosafety, human resources, training, technical support, and supplies with external quality assurance. Advantages are rapid turnaround time (72 h) for diagnosis of MDR-TB and early initiation of treatment will be possible.

Role of Blood-based, Immunological Tests

Although several blood-based tests are commercially available for TB, none of these are accurate. Antibody-based tests (IgG, IgM ELISA) are inaccurate and produce highly inconsistent results. The WHO issued a strong, negative recommendation against their use in 2011, and this is also reflected in the ISTC. Based on the WHO recommendations, the Indian Government banned serological antibody tests in 2012 and issued public notices about the ban. Various tests currently available are shown in Table 8.2. Table 8.3 shows various validated tests for the diagnosis of tuberculosis.

A comparative description of different diagnostic technologies as regards their requirements and costs are shown in Table 8.4.

TABLE 8.2

Various tests currently available

Type	Existing	Pipeline
Microscopy	• Ziehl-Neelsen staining • Conventional and light-emitting diode-based fluorescent microscopy	• TBDx (Signature Mapping Medical Sciences) automated system for smear microscopy that automatically loads and reads slides; needs optimization
Phenotypic culture	• Lowenstein-Jensen-based solid culture • Liquid culture (manual and automated)	• A colorimetric thin layer agar method to detect TB and screen for isoniazid, rifampicin, and ciprofloxacin resistance • The TREK Sensititre MYCOTB MIC—microtiter-plate-based liquid system for first and second DST
Molecular diagnosis	• Line probe assay • GeneXpert (feasibility ongoing for use under RNTCP)	• LAMP test—manual NAAT test at microscopy center level • TruNAAT test: micro-PCR handheld device—results in 30 min to 1 h • Genedrive (Epistem)—genotyping and sequencing test in a hand-held device; results within 1 h • B-SMART—detects TB and DR (first line) detection limit (<1,000) at present and being refined to <50 bacilli in sputum to be useful for smear negative cases

Continued

Continued

Various tests currently available

Type	Existing	Pipeline
Non-molecular tests	• Adenosine deaminase test for body fluids	• Breath analysis test—detection of volatile organic compounds • Alere TB LAM—urine LAM—lateral flow test–rule in TB with 71% sensitivity along with smear especially useful in HIV positive
Serological tests	• All currently available commercial serological tests banned for diagnosis of active TB	• MBio and FIND—developing a series of antigens for detection of active TB as a POC platform; field evaluation by late 2012 or 2013

TB, tuberculosis; DST, drug susceptibility testing; RNTCP, Revised National Tuberculosis Control Program; DR, drug resistant; POC, point-of-care; LAM, lipoarabinomannan; NAAT, Nucleic acid amplification testing; LAMP, Loop mediated isothermal amplification; PCR, polymerase chain reaction.

TABLE 8.3
Validated, World Health Organization-endorsed tests for active tuberculosis and drug susceptibility testing.

Test type or platform (reference for evidence)	Test description	Current validated commercial versions	WHO endorsed? (reference to policy)	Implemented by RNTCP?	Goal of testing (to detect)	Sensitivity	Specificity
Smear microscopy	Light-emitting diode fluorescence microscopy	Primo Star iLED™	Yes	Yes	Active TB	>60% (compared to culture)	98% (compared to culture)
Automated, CB-NAAT	CB-NAAT is a self-contained and fully automated technological platform that integrates sputum processing, DNA extraction and amplification, TB and MDR-TB diagnosis	Xpert MTB/RIF®	Yes	Yes	Active TB and DST	For active TB: >98% in smear-positive patients and 68% in smear-negative patients. For detecting drug resistance to rifampicin: 95%	For active TB: >98%. For detecting drug resistance to rifampicin: >98%

Continued

Continued

Validated, World Health Organization-endorsed tests for active tuberculosis and drug susceptibility testing.

Test type or platform (reference for evidence)	Test description	Current validated commercial versions	WHO endorsed? (reference to policy)	Implemented by RNTCP?	Goal of testing (to detect)	Sensitivity	Specificity
Liquid TB culture	Fully automated system for mycobacterial liquid culture and drug susceptibility testing	BACTEC MGIT® 960 BacT/ALERT® 3D	Yes	Yes	Active TB and DST	100% in smear-positive cases >75% in smear-negative cases	>99%
Line probe assays	Line probe assays for mutations that confer resistance to isoniazid and rifampicin	Hain Genotype MTBDRplus	Yes	Yes	Rapid DST for isoniazid and rifampicin resistance	98% for rifampicin resistance and 84% for isoniazid resistance	99% for rifampicin resistance and 99% for isoniazid

WHO, World Health Organization; RNTCP, Revised National Tuberculosis Control Program; TB, tuberculosis; CB-NAAT, cartridge-based nucleic acid amplification test; MDR-TB, multidrug-resistant tuberculosis; DNA, deoxyribonucleic acid; DST, drug susceptibility testing; MTB, *Mycobacterium tuberculosis*, RIF, rifampicin.

TABLE 8.4

Training, infrastructure, equipment, and consumables requirements for each type of test				
Technology	*Training*	*Infrastructure*	*Equipment*	*Consumables*
Liquid culture and DST	Extensive (3 weeks)	Biosafety level: 3	High	High
Strip speciation	Minimal (1 day)	Biosafety level: 3	Low	Medium
Molecular line probe assay	Moderate (3 days)	Biosafety level: 2–3	High	Low
Light-emitting diode fluorescence microscopy	Moderate	Basic laboratory	Medium	Low
Noncommercial culture and DST methods	Extensive	Biosafety level: 2–3	Low	Medium
Automated detection and MDR screening	Minimal	Basic laboratory	High	High

Basic laboratory: no specialized biosafety equipment required.
Biosafety level 2: specialized biosafety equipment required, such as biosafety cabinet.
Biosafety level 3: biosafety cabinet and other primary safety equipment required; controlled ventilation system that maintains a directional airflow into the laboratory required.
DST, drug susceptibility testing; MDR, multidrug resistant.

DIAGNOSIS OF LATENT TUBERCULOSIS INFECTION

Two tests are available currently: the TST (performed using Mantoux technique) and the IGRA. Evidence suggests that both TST and IGRA are acceptable but imperfect tests. They represent indirect markers of *M. tuberculosis* exposure and indicate a cellular immune response to *M. tuberculosis*. Neither test can accurately differentiate between latent TB infections (LTBI) and active TB, distinguish reactivation from reinfection or resolve the various stages within the spectrum of *M. tuberculosis* infection. In addition, both have reduced sensitivity in immunocompromised patients (e.g., HIV-infected). Both tests have low predictive value for progression to active TB. To maximize the positive predictive value of existing tests, LTBI screening is reserved only for those who are at sufficiently high risk of progressing to disease to outweigh the known harms of LTBI treatment. Most importantly, both TST and IGRAs should not be used for the diagnosis of active TB in high endemic settings like India. In children, these tests may have some value as a test for infection, in addition to chest X-rays, symptoms, history of contact, and other microbiological investigations (e.g., gastric juice AFB and Xpert MTB/RIF).

Various diagnostic technologies with their sensitivities are shown in Figure 8.10. The recommended choice of different diagnostic tests by the RNTCP is shown in Table 8.5.

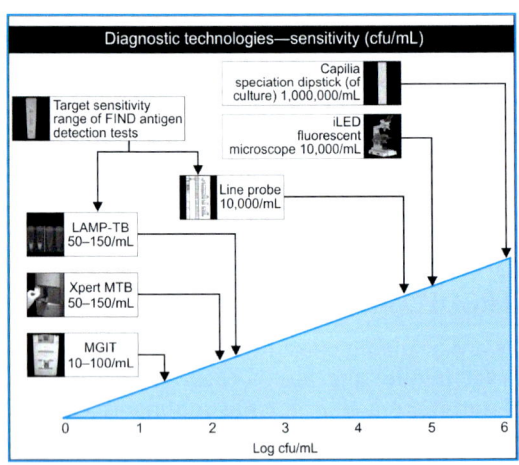

MTB, *Mycobacterium tuberculosis*; LAMP, Loop mediated isothermal amplification; TB, tuberculosis; MGIT, mycobacteria growth indicator tube.

Figure 8.10 Various diagnostic technologies with their sensitivities.

Laboratory Diagnosis of Tuberculosis

Figure 8.11 shows various settings where these tests can be and should be undertaken.

TABLE 8.5

Choice of diagnostic technology of drug-resistant tuberculosis under Revised National Tuberculosis Control Program	
Multidrug-resistant diagnostic technology	*Choice*
Molecular DST (e.g., LPA DST or CB-NAAT)	First
Liquid culture isolation and LPA DST	Second
Solid culture isolation and LPA DST	Third
Liquid culture isolation and liquid DST	Fourth
Solid culture isolation and DST	Fifth

DST, drug susceptibility testing; LPA, line probe assay; CB-NAAT, cartridge-based nucleic acid amplification test.

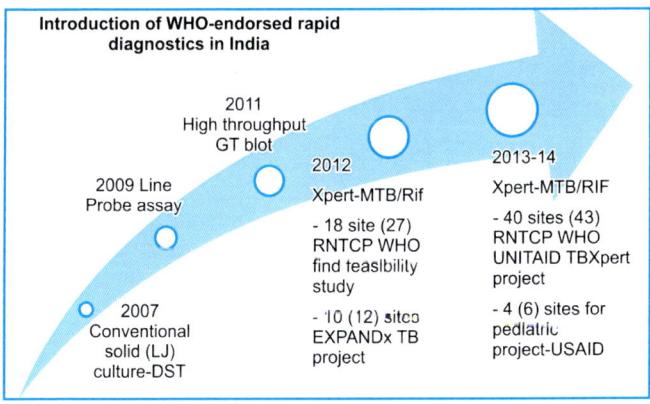

WHO, World Health organization; RNTCP, Revised National Tuberculosis Control Program; USAID, United States Agency for International Development; DST, drug susceptibility testing; MTB, *Mycobacterium tuberculosis*; RIF, rifampicin.

Figure 8.11 WHO endorsed rapid diagnostics in India.

Clinic Consult Pulmonology: Tuberculosis

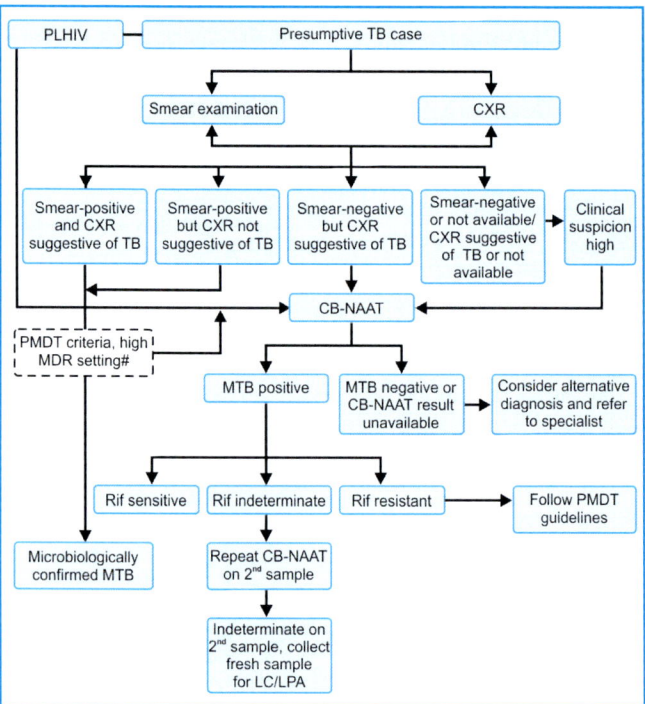

CB-NAAT, cartridge-based nucleic acid amplification test; CXR, chest X-ray; MTB, Mycobacterium tuberculosis; PMDT, program management of drug resistant tuberculosis; DD, differential diagnosis; Rif, rifampicin; LC, liquid culture; LPA, line probe assay; PLHIV, people living with human immunodeficiency virus.

#Settings identified as per global guidelines and the program data.

Figure 8.12 The diagnostic algorithm for tuberculosis in India.

The algorithm used for diagnosis of tuberculosis in India as practiced now is shown in Figure 8.12. However, the new strategic plan document developed now in 2017 has a different approach now with focus on active case finding and CBNAAT test and chest radiology for the diagnosis have importance.

Laboratory Diagnosis of Tuberculosis

The algorithm includes pulmonary, extra-pulmonary, pediatric tuberculosis as well as that in association with HIV. They will be available in the Technical Operational Guidelines in the RNTCP website.

> **KEY MESSAGE**
>
> ❏ A number of diagnostics are available now for tuberculosis. The need of the hour is to get tools and equipments focused on tuberculosis.

SUGGESTED READINGS

1. Boehme CC, Nabeta P, Hillemann D, Nicol MP, Shenai S, Krapp F, et al. Rapid molecular detection of tuberculosis and rifampin resistance. N Engl J Med. 2010;363:1005-15.
2. Cruciani M, Scarparo C, Malena M, Bosco O, Serpelloni G, Mengoli C. Meta-analysis of BACTEC MGIT 960 and BACTEC 460 TB, with or without solid media, for detection of mycobacteria. J Clin Microbiol. 2004;42:2321-5.
3. Grenier J, Pinto L, Nair D, Steingart K, Dowdy D, Ramsay A, Pai M. Widespread use of serological tests for tuberculosis: data from 22 high-burden countries. Eur Respir J. 2012;39:502-5.
4. Horne DJ, Pinto LM, Arentz M, Lin SY, Desmond E, Flores LL, et al. Diagnostic accuracy and reproducibility of WHO-endorsed phenotypic drug susceptibility testing methods for first-line and second-line anti-tuberculosis drugs: a systematic review and meta-analysis. J Clin Microbiol. 2013;51:393-401.
5. Kik SV, Qin ZZ, Pai M. Optimal diagnosis: how early and improved diagnosis can help prevent TB transmission. Clinical Insights by Future Medicine. 2013:7-32.
6. Pai M, Denkinger C, Kik SV, Rangaka MX, Zwerling A, Oxlade O, et al. Interferon-gamma release assays for the detection of Mycobacterium tuberculosis infection. Clin Microbiol Rev. 2014;27:1-18.
7. Pai M. Diagnosis of pulmonary tuberculosis: recent advances. J Indian Med Assoc. 2013;111:332-336.

8. Pai M. Promoting affordable and quality tuberculosis testing in India. J Lab Physicians. 2013;5:1-4.
9. Rangaka MX, Wilkinson KA, Glynn JR, Ling D, Menzies D, Mwansa-Kambafwile J, et al. Predictive value of interferon-gamma release assays for incident active tuberculosis: a systematic review and meta-analysis. Lancet Infect Dis. 2012;12:45-55.
10. Revised National TB Control Programme Manual of Standard Operating Procedures (SOPs) Culture of Mycobacterium tuberculosis and Drug Susceptibility Testing on solid Medium. Revised National Tuberculosis Control Programme Central TB Division. Ministry of Health & Family Welfare: New Delhi; 2009.
11. Reza LW, Satyanarayna S, Enarson DA, Kumar AM, Sagili K, Kumar S, et al. LED-Fluorescence Microscopy for Diagnosis of Pulmonary Tuberculosis under Programmatic Conditions in India. PLoS One. 2013;8(10):e75566.
12. Sreeramareddy CT, Qin ZZ, Satyanarayana S, Subbaraman R, Pai M. Delays in diagnosis and treatment of pulmonary tuberculosis in India: a systematic review. Int J Tuberc Lung Dis. 2014;18:255-66.
13. Steingart K, Sohn H, Schiller I, Kloda LA, Boehme CC, Pai M, Dendukuri N. et al. Xpert® MTB/RIF assay for pulmonary tuberculosis and rifampicin resistance in adults. Cochrane Database Syst Rev. 2013;1:CD009593.
14. Steingart KR, Flores LL, Dendukuri N, Schiller I, Laal S, Ramsay A, et al. Commercial serological tests for the diagnosis of active pulmonary and extrapulmonary tuberculosis: an updated systematic review and meta-analysis. PLoS Med. 2011;8(8):e1001062.
15. Steingart KR, Henry M, Ng V, Hopewell PC, Ramsay A, Cunningham J, et al. Fluorescence versus conventional sputum smear microscopy for tuberculosis: a systematic review. Lancet Infect Dis. 2006;6:570-81.
16. Steingart KR, Ramsay A, Pai M. Optimizing sputum smear microscopy for the diagnosis of pulmonary tuberculosis. Expert Rev Anti Infect Ther. 2007;5:327-31.
17. World Health Organization. Fluorescent light-emitting diode (LED) microscopy for diagnosis of tuberculosis: policy statement. 2011. Available from: http://whqlibdoc.who.int/publications/2011/9789241501613_eng.pdf.
18. World Health Organization. Policy statement. Molecular line probe assays for rapid screening of patients at risk of multidrug-resistant tuberculosis (MDR-TB). 2008. Available from: http://www.who.int/tb/laboratory/policy_statements/en/index.html.

19. World Health Organization. Policy statement: Commercial serodiagnostic tests for diagnosis of tuberculosis. 2011. Available from: http://www.who.int/tb/laboratory/roadmap_xpert_mtb_rif_rev23dec2010.pdf.
20. World Health Organization. Policy update: automated real-time nucleic acid amplification technology for rapid and simultaneous detection of tuberculosis and rifampicin resistance: Xpert MTB/RIF system for the diagnosis of pulmonary and extrapulmonary TB in adults and children. 2013. Available from: http://www.stoptb.org/wg/gli/assets/documents/WHO%20Policy%20Statement%20on%20Xpert%20MTB-RIF%202013%20pre%20publication%2022102013.pdf.
21. World Health Organization. The use of liquid medium for culture and DST. Vol 2008. World Health Organization: Geneva; 2007.
22. World Health Organization. Use of tuberculosis interferon-gamma release assays (IGRAs) in low- and middle-income countries: policy statement. 2011.

CHAPTER 9

Antituberculosis Drugs

INTRODUCTION

Antituberculosis (anti-TB) drugs are classified into five groups based on evidence of efficacy, potency, drug class, and experience of use. All first line anti-TB drug names have a standard three-letter and/or a single-letter abbreviation. First line anti-TB drugs (group 1) are currently recommended in a four-drug combination for the treatment of drug susceptible TB. Second line anti-TB drugs (groups 2, 3, and 4) are reserved for drug-resistant TB. Third line anti-TB drugs (group 5) have unclear efficacy or undefined roles.

- First line anti-TB drugs
  - Group 1: oral—isoniazid (H/Inh), rifampicin/rifampin (R/Rif), pyrazinamide (Z/Pza), ethambutol (E/Emb), rifapentine (P/Rpt), or rifabutin (Rfb)
- Second line anti-TB drugs
  - Group 2: injectable aminoglycosides—streptomycin (S/Stm), kanamycin (Km), amikacin (Amk). Injectable polypeptides—capreomycin (Cm), viomycin (Vim)
  - Group 3: oral and injectable fluoroquinolones—ciprofloxacin (Cfx), levofloxacin (Lfx), moxifloxacin (Mfx), ofloxacin (Ofx), gatifloxacin (Gfx)
  - Group 4: oral—para-aminosalicylic acid (Pas), cycloserine (Dcs), terizidone (Trd), ethionamide (Eto), prothionamide (Pto), thioacetazone (Thz), linezolid (Lzd)

Antituberculosis Drugs

- Third line anti-TB drugs
  - Group 5: clofazimine (Cfz), linezolid (Lzd), amoxicillin plus clavulanate (Amx/Clv), imipenem plus cilastatin (Ipm/Cln), clarithromycin (Clr). WHO has recently recommended another classification, particularly those used for MDR and XDR treatment. They will be discussed subsequently.

The five basic or "first line" TB drugs are isoniazid, rifampicin, pyrazinamide, ethambutol, and streptomycin. These are the TB drugs that generally have the greatest activity against TB bacteria and are core to any TB drug treatment program. These TB drugs are particularly used for someone with active TB disease who has not had TB drug treatment before. All the other TB drugs are generally referred to as "second line" or reserve TB drugs.

There are also newer drugs developed recently with ten compounds those have progressed into the clinical development pipeline, including six new compounds specifically developed for TB like bedaquiline (TMC207-C210), delamanid (OPC-67683), and pretomanid (PA-824 and TBA-354).

ISONIAZID

Isoniazid, is the hydrazide of isonicotinic acid. It is highly bactericidal against replicating tubercle bacilli. It is rapidly absorbed and diffuses readily into all fluids and tissues. The plasma half-life, which is genetically determined, varies from less than 1 hour in fast acetylators to more than 3 hours in slow acetylators. Isoniazid is largely excreted in the urine within 24 hours, mostly as inactive metabolites. It is normally taken orally but may be administered intramuscularly or intravenously to critically ill patients. The dose in adults is 5 mg/kg (4–6 mg/kg) daily, maximum 300 mg; 10 mg/kg (8–12 mg/kg) three times weekly, maximum 900 mg. Contraindications are known hypersensitivity and active, unstable hepatic disease (with jaundice). Clinical monitoring (and liver function tests, if possible) should be performed during treatment of patients with preexisting liver disease. Patients at risk of peripheral neuropathy, as a result of malnutrition, chronic alcohol dependence, human immunodeficiency virus (HIV) infection, pregnancy, breastfeeding, renal failure, or diabetes, should additionally receive pyridoxine (10 mg daily). In the community of low health standard, pyridoxine should be offered routinely; some guidelines recommend a dose of 25 mg/day to prevent peripheral neuropathy. For established peripheral neuropathy, pyridoxine should be given at a larger dose of 50–75 mg daily.

Since isoniazid interacts with anticonvulsants used for epilepsy, it may be necessary to reduce the dosage of these drugs during treatment with isoniazid. If possible, serum concentrations of phenytoin and carbamazepine should be measured in patients receiving isoniazid with or without rifampicin. Isoniazid is not known to be harmful in pregnancy. Pyridoxine supplementation is recommended for all pregnant (or breastfeeding) women taking isoniazid.

Adverse Effects

Isoniazid is generally well tolerated at recommended doses. Systemic or cutaneous hypersensitivity reactions occasionally occur during the first weeks of treatment. Sleepiness or lethargy can be managed by reassurance or adjustment of the timing of administration. The risk of peripheral neuropathy is excluded if vulnerable patients receive daily supplements of pyridoxine. Other less common forms of neurological disturbance, including optic neuritis, toxic psychosis, and generalized convulsions, can develop in susceptible individuals, particularly in the later stages of treatment, and occasionally necessitate the withdrawal of isoniazid. Symptomatic hepatitis is an uncommon but potentially serious reaction that can usually be averted by prompt withdrawal of treatment. More often, however, an asymptomatic rise in serum concentrations of hepatic transaminases at the outset of treatment is of no clinical significance and usually resolves spontaneously as treatment continues. A lupus-like syndrome, pellagra, anemia, and arthralgias are other rare adverse effects. Monoamine poisoning has been reported to occur after ingestion of foods and beverages with high monoamine content, but this is also rare.

Drug Interactions

Isoniazid inhibits the metabolism of certain drugs, which can increase their plasma concentrations to the point of toxicity. Rifampicin, however, has the opposite effect for many of these drugs. For example, the available data indicate that administering both rifampicin and isoniazid causes a reduction in plasma levels of phenytoin and diazepam. Isoniazid may increase the toxicity of carbamazepine, benzodiazepines metabolized by oxidation (such as triazolam), acetaminophen, valproate, serotonergic antidepressants, disulfiram, warfarin, and theophylline. Overdosage of isoniazid will cause nausea, vomiting, dizziness, blurred vision, and slurring of speech occur within 30 minutes to 3 hours of overdosage. Massive poisoning results in coma preceded by respiratory depression and stupor. Severe intractable seizures may occur. Emesis and gastric lavage, activated charcoal, antiepileptics, and intravenous sodium bicarbonate can be of value if instituted within a few hours of ingestion. Subsequently, hemodialysis may be of value. High doses of pyridoxine must be administered to prevent seizures.

RIFAMPICIN

It is a semisynthetic derivative of rifamycin and is a complex macrocyclic antibiotic that inhibits ribonucleic acid synthesis in a broad range of microbial pathogens. It has bactericidal action and a potent sterilizing effect against tubercle bacilli in both cellular and extracellular locations. It is lipid-soluble. Following oral administration, it is rapidly absorbed and distributed throughout the cellular tissues and body fluids; if the meninges are inflamed, significant amounts enter the cerebrospinal fluid. A single dose of 600 mg produces a peak serum concentration of about 10 μg/mL in 2–4 hours, which subsequently decays with a half-life of 2–3 hours. It is extensively recycled in the enterohepatic circulation, and metabolites formed by deacetylation in the liver are eventually excreted in the feces. Since resistance readily develops, rifampicin must always be administered in combination with other effective antimycobacterial agents.

Rifampicin should preferably be given at least 30 minutes before meals, since absorption is reduced when it is taken with food. However, this may not be clinically significant, and food can reduce intolerance to drugs. It is also available for intravenous administration in critically ill patients. The dose in adults is 10 mg/kg (8–12 mg/kg) daily or 3 times weekly—maximum 600 mg. It is contraindicated in known hypersensitivity to rifamycins and active, unstable hepatic disease (with jaundice). Serious immunological reactions resulting in renal impairment, hemolysis, or thrombocytopenia are reported in patients who resume taking rifampicin after a prolonged lapse of treatment. In this rare situation, rifampicin should be immediately and permanently withdrawn. Clinical monitoring (and liver function tests, if possible) should be performed during treatment of all patients with preexisting liver disease, who are at increased risk of further liver damage. Patients should be warned that treatment may cause reddish coloration of all body secretions (urine, tears, saliva, sweat, semen, and sputum), and that contact lenses and clothing may be irreversibly stained.

In pregnancy, vitamin K should be administered at birth to the infant of a mother taking rifampicin because of the risk of postnatal hemorrhage.

Adverse Effects

Rifampicin is well tolerated by most patients at currently recommended doses, but may cause gastrointestinal reactions (abdominal pain, nausea, vomiting) and pruritus with or without rash. Other adverse effects [fever, influenza-like (flu-like) syndrome, and thrombocytopenia] are more likely to occur with intermittent administration. Exfoliative dermatitis is more frequent in HIV-positive TB patients. Temporary oliguria, dyspnea, and hemolytic anemia have also been reported in patients taking the drug three times weekly; these reactions usually subside if the regimen is changed to daily dosage. Moderate rises in serum concentrations of bilirubin and transaminases, which are common at the outset of treatment, are often transient and without clinical significance. However, dose-related hepatitis can occur and is potentially fatal; it is therefore important not to exceed the maximum recommended daily dose of 600 mg.

Drug Interactions

Rifampicin induces hepatic enzymes, and may increase the dosage requirements of drugs metabolized in the liver, including:

Clinic Consult Pulmonology: Tuberculosis

- Anti-infectives (certain antiretroviral drugs, mefloquine, azole antifungal agents, clarithromycin, erythromycin, doxycycline, atovaquone, and chloramphenicol)
- Hormone therapy including ethinylestradiol, norethindrone, tamoxifen, and levothyroxine
- Methadone
- Warfarin
- Cyclosporine
- Corticosteroids
- Anticonvulsants (including phenytoin)
- Cardiovascular agents including digoxin (in patients with renal insufficiency), digitoxin, verapamil, nifedipine, diltiazem, propranolol, metoprorol, enalapril, losartan, quinidine, mexiletine, tocainide, and propafenone
- Theophylline
- Sulfonylurea hypoglycemics
- Hypolipidemics including simvastatin and fluvastatin
- Nortriptyline, haloperidol, quetiapine, benzodiazepines (including diazepam, triazolam), zolpidem, and buspirone.

Since rifampicin reduces the effectiveness of oral contraceptives, women should be advised to choose between one of two options for contraception. Following consultation with a clinician, the patient may use an oral contraceptive pill containing a higher dose of estrogen (50 μg). Alternatively, a nonhormonal method of contraception may be used throughout rifampicin treatment and for at least one month subsequently.

Current antiretroviral drugs (non-nucleoside reverse transcriptase inhibitors and protease inhibitors) interact with rifampicin. This may result in ineffectiveness of antiretroviral drugs, ineffective treatment of TB or an increased risk of drug toxicity.

Biliary excretion of radiocontrast media and sulfobromophthalein sodium may be reduced and microbiological assays for folic acid and vitamin B12 disturbed.

Overdosage

Gastric lavage may be of value if undertaken within a few hours of ingestion. Very large doses of rifampicin may depress central nervous function. There is no specific antidote and treatment is supportive.

PYRAZINAMIDE

Pyrazinamide is a synthetic analog of nicotinamide and is only weakly bactericidal against *M. tuberculosis* but has potent sterilizing activity, particularly in the relatively acidic intracellular environment of macrophages and in areas of acute inflammation. It is highly effective during the first 2 months of treatment while acute inflammatory changes persist. Its use has enabled treatment regimens to be shortened and the risk of relapse to be reduced.

It is readily absorbed from the gastrointestinal tract and is rapidly distributed throughout all tissues and fluids. Peak plasma concentrations are attained in 2 hours and the plasma half-life is about 10 hours. It is metabolized mainly in the liver and excreted largely in the urine. The drug is administered orally. In adults (usually for the first 2 or 3 months of TB treatment): 25 mg/kg (20–30 mg/kg) daily; or 35 mg/kg (30–40 mg/kg) 3 times weekly. It is contraindicated in known hypersensitivity, active, unstable hepatic disease (with jaundice), and porphyria. Patients with diabetes should be carefully monitored since blood glucose concentrations may become labile. Gout may be exacerbated. Clinical monitoring (and liver function tests, if possible) should be performed during treatment of patients with preexisting liver disease. In patients with renal failure, pyrazinamide should be administered three times per week rather than daily. Although detailed teratogenicity data are not available, pyrazinamide can probably be used safely during pregnancy.

Adverse Effects

Pyrazinamide may cause gastrointestinal intolerance. Hypersensitivity reactions are rare, but some patients complain of slight flushing of the skin. Moderate rises in serum transaminase concentrations are common during the early phases of treatment. Severe hepatotoxicity is rare. As a result of inhibition of renal tubular secretion, a degree of hyperuricemia usually occurs, but this is often asymptomatic. Gout requiring treatment with allopurinol occasionally develops. Arthralgia, particularly of the shoulders, may occur and is responsive to simple analgesics (especially aspirin). Both hyperuricemia and arthralgia may be reduced by prescribing regimens with intermittent administration of pyrazinamide. Rare adverse events include sideroblastic anemia and photosensitive dermatitis. Little has been recorded on the management of pyrazinamide overdose. Acute liver damage and hyperuricemia have been reported. Treatment is essentially symptomatic. Emesis and gastric lavage may be of value if undertaken within a few hours of ingestion. There is no specific antidote and treatment is supportive.

STREPTOMYCIN

Streptomycin is an aminoglycoside antibiotic derived from *S. griseus* that is used in the treatment of TB and sensitive Gram-negative infections. Streptomycin is not absorbed from the gastrointestinal tract but, after intramuscular administration, it diffuses readily into the extracellular component of most body tissues and attains bactericidal concentrations, particularly in tuberculous cavities. Little normally enters the cerebrospinal fluid, although penetration increases when the meninges are inflamed. The plasma half-life, which is normally 2–3 hours, is considerably extended in the newborn, the elderly, and patients with severe renal impairment. Streptomycin is excreted unchanged in the urine.

Antituberculosis Drugs

Streptomycin must be administered by deep intramuscular injection. It is also available for intravenous administration. The dose in adults is 15 mg/kg (12–18 mg/kg) daily, or 2 or 3 times weekly; maximum daily dose is 1,000 mg. Patients aged over 60 years may not be able to tolerate more than 500–750 mg daily, so some guidelines recommend reducing the dose to 10 mg/kg per day for patients in this age group. Patients weighing less than 50 kg may not tolerate doses above 500–750 mg daily.

The drug is contraindicated in known hypersensitivity, auditory nerve impairment, myasthenia gravis, and pregnancy.

Precautions

Hypersensitivity reactions are rare; if they do occur (usually during the first weeks of treatment), streptomycin should be withdrawn immediately. Once fever and skin rash have resolved, desensitization may be attempted. Both the elderly and patients with renal impairment are vulnerable to dose-related toxic effects resulting from accumulation. Streptomycin should be used with caution in patients with renal insufficiency, because of the increased risk of nephrotoxicity and ototoxicity. The dose should be maintained at 12–15 mg/kg but at a reduced frequency of 2–3 times per week. Where possible, serum levels should be monitored periodically and dosage adjusted appropriately to ensure that plasma concentrations, as measured when the next dose is due, do not exceed 4 µg mL. Protective gloves should be worn when streptomycin injections are administered to avoid sensitization dermatitis. Streptomycin should not be used in pregnancy; it crosses the placenta and can cause auditory nerve impairment and nephrotoxicity in the fetus.

Adverse Effects

Streptomycin injections are painful. Rash, induration, or sterile abscesses can form at injection sites. Numbness and tingling around the mouth (circum-oral parasthesia) occur immediately after injection. Cutaneous hypersensitivity reactions can occur. Impairment of vestibular function is uncommon with currently recommended doses. Hearing loss is less common than vertigo. Manifestations of damage to the 8th cranial (auditory) nerve include ringing in the ears, ataxia, vertigo, and deafness; damage usually occurs in the first 2 months of treatment and is reversible if the dosage is reduced or the drug is stopped. Streptomycin is less nephrotoxic than other aminoglycoside antibiotics. If urinary output falls, albuminuria occurs or tubular casts are detected in the urine, streptomycin should be stopped and renal function should be evaluated. Hemolytic anemia, aplastic anemia, agranulocytosis, thrombocytopenia, and lupoid reactions are rare adverse effects. Other ototoxic or nephrotoxic drugs should not be administered to patients receiving streptomycin. These include other aminoglycoside antibiotics, amphotericin B, cefalosporins, etacrynic acid, cyclosporin, cisplatin, furosemide, and vancomycin. Streptomycin may potentiate the effect of neuromuscular blocking agents administered during anesthesia. Hemodialysis can be beneficial in case of over dosage. There is no specific antidote and treatment is supportive.

ETHAMBUTOL

It is a synthetic congener of 1,2-ethanediamine, and is active against *M. tuberculosis*, *M. bovis,* and some nonspecific mycobacteria. It is used in combination with other anti-TB drugs to prevent or delay the emergence of resistant strains. It is readily absorbed from the gastrointestinal tract. Plasma concentrations peak in 2–4 hours and decay with a half-life of 3–4 hours. Ethambutol is excreted in the urine both unchanged and as inactive hepatic metabolites. About 20%

is excreted unchanged in the feces. The drug is administered orally to adults in a dosage of 15 mg/kg (15–20 mg/kg) daily or 30 mg/kg (25–35 mg/kg) three times weekly. Dosage must always be carefully calculated on a weight basis to avoid toxicity, and the dose or the dosing interval should be adjusted in patients with impaired renal function (creatinine clearance <70 mL/min). If creatinine clearance is less than 30 mL/min, ethambutol should be administered three times per week. It is contraindicated in known hypersensitivity and preexisting optic neuritis from any cause. Patients should be advised to discontinue treatment immediately and to report to a clinician if their sight or perception of color deteriorates. Ocular examination is recommended before and during treatment. Whenever possible, renal function should be assessed before treatment. Plasma ethambutol concentration should be monitored if creatinine clearance is less than 30 mL/min. Ethambutol is not known to be harmful in pregnancy.

Adverse Effects

Dose-dependent optic neuritis can result in impairment of visual acuity and color vision in one or both eyes. Early changes are usually reversible, but blindness can occur if treatment is not discontinued promptly. Ocular toxicity is rare when ethambutol is used for 2–3 months at recommended doses. Signs of peripheral neuritis occasionally develop in the legs. Other rare adverse events include generalized cutaneous reaction, arthralgia and, very rarely, hepatitis. Emesis and gastric lavage may be of value in case of over dosage if undertaken within a few hours of ingestion. Subsequently, dialysis may be of value. There is no specific antidote and treatment is supportive. The dosage of various anti-tubercular drugs is shown in Table 9.1.

TABLE 9.1

Recommended doses for first line antituberculosis drugs for adults (World Health Organization, 2010)

Drugs	Dose recommended			
	If used daily		If intermittent therapy (three times per week)	
	Dose and range in mg/kg body weight	Maximum dose (mg)	Dose and range in mg/kg body weight	Daily maximum dose (mg)
Isoniazid	5 (4–6)	300	10 (8–12)	900
Rifampicin	10 (8–12)	600	10 (8–12)	600
Pyrazinamide	25 (20–30)	–	35 (30–40)	–
Ethambutol	15 (15–20)	–	30 (25–35)	–
Streptomycin*	15 (12–18)	–	15 (12–18)	1,000

*Patients aged over 60 years may not be able to tolerate more than 500–750 mg daily, so some guidelines recommend reduction of the dose to 10 mg/kg per day in patients in this age group. Patients weighing less than 50 kg may not tolerate doses above 500–750 mg daily.

Antituberculosis Drugs

STANDARD REGIMENS

- It is advised to use standardized treatment rather than individualized prescription of drugs, particularly in program conditions
- This approach avoids errors in prescription which will avoid the risk of development of drug resistance; enables estimating drug needs, purchasing, distribution, and monitoring are facilitated; better staff training; costs are reduced; helps in maintaining a regular drug supply when patients move from one area to another; and outcome evaluation is convenient and results are comparable.

New Patient

The frequency of therapy ideally should be daily which is optimal. However, other alternatives are recommended (Tables 9.2 to 9.4).

Standard Regimens for Previously Treated Patients

- As the chances of development of multidrug-resistant TB (MDR-TB) is very high in this group, they are to be tested for exclusion of MDR-TB

TABLE 9.2

Standard treatment for new patients (presumed or known to have drug susceptible tuberculosis)	
Intensive phase (2 months)	*Continuation phase (4 months)*
HRZE	HR

H, isoniazid; R, rifampicin; Z, pyrazinamide; E, ethambutol.
Note: World Health Organization no longer recommends omission of ethambutol during the intensive phase of treatment for patients with noncavitary, smear-negative pulmonary or extrapulmonary tuberculosis who are known to be human immunodeficiency virus-negative. In tuberculous meningitis, ethambutol should be replaced by streptomycin.

Clinic Consult Pulmonology: Tuberculosis

TABLE 9.3

Dosing frequency for new tuberculosis patients		
Dose frequency		
Intensive phase	*Continuation phase*	*Comments*
Daily	Daily	Ideal
Daily	Three times per week	Acceptable alternative for any new tuberculosis patient receiving directly observed therapy
Three times per week	Three times per week	Acceptable alternative provided that the patient is receiving directly observed therapy and is not living with HIV or living in an HIV prevalent setting

HIV, human immunodeficiency virus.
Note: Daily (rather than three times weekly) intensive phase therapy may help to prevent acquired drug resistance in tuberculosis patients starting treatment with isoniazid resistance.

TABLE 9.4

Standard regimens for new tuberculosis patients in settings where the level of isoniazid resistance among new tuberculosis cases is high and isoniazid susceptibility testing is not done or results are not available before the continuation phase begins	
Intensive phase treatment	*Continuation phase*
2 months of HRZE	4 months of HRE

H, isoniazid; R, rifampicin; Z, pyrazinamide; E, ethambutol.
Note: The continuation phase contains three drugs including additional ethambutol.

- The RNTCP of India has now accepted and advocates the regimen mentioned in Table 9.4
- It is recommended that specimens for culture and drug susceptibility testing (DST) should be obtained from all previously treated TB patients at or before the start of treatment. DST should be performed for at least isoniazid and rifampicin.

DRUG REGIMENS USED IN REVISED NATIONAL TUBERCULOSIS CONTROL PROGRAM

The Revised National Tuberculosis Control Program (RNTCP) of India uses intermittent therapy (thrice weekly) since its inception and has the two categories of treatment (Table 9.5).

The program uses short course chemotherapy given intermittently—thrice weekly under direct observation for both pulmonary and extrapulmonary TB patients. If the sputum smear is positive after 2 months of treatment, the intensive phase of four drugs (isoniazid, rifampicin, pyrazinamide, and ethambutol) is continued for another 1 month and sputum examined after the completion of the extension of intensive phase. Irrespective of the sputum results after this extension of the intensive phase, 4 months of the continuation phase is started. If the sputum smear is positive after 5 or more months of treatment, the patient is declared as a "failure" and is placed on the "previously treated" treatment regimen afresh, and sputum sent for culture and DST to a certified RNTCP culture and DST laboratory. With introduction of cartridge-based nucleic acid amplification test (CB-NAAT), this is the preferred mode of testing.

TABLE 9.5

The Revised National Tuberculosis Control Program categories of treatment
Category I
• For all the "new" pulmonary (smear positive and negative), extrapulmonary, and other tuberculosis patients, regimen is: 2H3R3Z3E3/4H3R3 (total duration 6 months)
Category II
• All "relapses, treatment after default, failures, and others" are treated with the regimen for previously-treated cases: 2S3H3R3Z3E3/1H3R3Z3E3/5H3R3E3 (total duration 8 months)

E, ethambutol; H, isoniazid; R, rifampicin; S, streptomycin; Z, pyrazinamide.

All those patients who have received anti-TB treatment for more than 1 month earlier are classified as "previously treated". These patients are at a higher risk of having drug resistance. The intensive phase consists of 2 months of isoniazid, rifampicin, pyrazinamide, ethambutol, and streptomycin, followed by 1 month of isoniazid, rifampicin, pyrazinamide, and ethambutol (Table 9.6). Patient is subjected for follow-up sputum examination at the end of 3 months. If the sputum smear is positive at the end of 3 months of treatment, the intensive phase is extended for another 1 month. Irrespective of the sputum results at the end of the extended intensive phase, continuation phase is started. If the sputum remains positive at the end of the extended intensive phase, sputum is sent to a certified RNTCP culture and DST laboratory for culture and DST. The continuation phase consists of 5 months of isoniazid, rifampicin, and ethambutol given thrice a week on alternate days. The CB-NAAT now is the preferred mode of identification for all previously treated cases (category II cases).

The RNTCP regimen used so far was basically intermittent as shown in Table 9.5. However, currently the program has changed over to daily therapy as shown in Table 9.4. Under RNTCP, drugs are supplied in patient-wise boxes (PWB) containing the full course of treatment and packaged in blister packs. The PWB has a color code indicating the two regimens—red for "new" and blue for "previously treated". In each PWB, there are two pouches, one for the intensive phase and one for the continuation phase, for operational convenience. The dosage strengths are as follows: isoniazid 600 mg, rifampicin 450 mg, pyrazinamide 1,500 mg, ethambutol 1,200 mg, and streptomycin 750 mg. Patients who weigh 60 kg or more receive additional rifampicin 150 mg. Patients who are more than 50 years old receive streptomycin 500 mg. Patients who weigh less than 30 kg, receive drugs as per pediatric weight band boxes according to body weight.

Antituberculosis Drugs

TABLE 9.6

Standard regimens for previously treated patients depending on the availability of routine drug susceptibility testing to guide the therapy of individual retreatment patients		
Drug susceptibility testing (DST)	Likelihood of multidrug resistant (MDR; patient characteristics*)	
Routinely available for previously treated patients	High (failure#)	Medium or low (relapse, default)
Rapid molecular-based method	MDR results available in 1–2 days confirm or exclude MDR to guide the choice of regimen	
Conventional method	• While awaiting DST results:[†] empirical multidrug resistant regimen • Regimen should be modified once DST results are available	• 2HRZES/1HRZE/5HRE • Regimen should be modified once DST results are available
None (interim)	• Empirical MDR regimen • Regimen should be modified once DST results or DRS data are available	• 2HRZES/1HRZE/5HRE for full course of treatment • Regimen should be modified once DST results or DRS data are available

H, isoniazid; R, rifampicin; Z, pyrazinamide; E, ethambutol; S, streptomycin; MDR, multidrug resistant; DRS, drug resistance surveillance.

*The assumption that failure patients have a high likelihood of MDR (and relapse or defaulting patients a medium likelihood) may need to be modified according to the level of MDR in these patient registration groups.

#And other patients in groups with high levels of MDR like patients who develop active TB after known contact with a patient with documented MDR-TB. Patients who are relapsing or returning after defaulting from their second or subsequent course of treatment probably also have a high likelihood of MDR.

[†]Regimen may be modified once DST results are available (up to 2–3 months after the start of treatment).

Caution: In the standard regimens, the 8-month retreatment regimen should not be "augmented" by a fluoroquinolone or an injectable second line drug; this will jeopardize second line drugs that are critical treatment options for MDR patients. Second line drugs should be used only for MDR regimens and only if quality assured drugs can be provided by directly observed treatment for the whole course of therapy. In addition, there must be laboratory capacity for cultures to monitor treatment response, as well as a system for detecting and treating adverse reactions before embarking on MDR-TB treatment.

Streptomycin is absolutely contraindicated during entire pregnancy. Breastfeeding can be continued even when mother is on treatment for TB but mother should continue to practice cough hygiene. Child should be administered preventive chemoprophylaxis as per guidelines.

In rare and exceptional situations, non-DOTS, treatment (with a self-administered non-rifampicin containing regimen) may be needed in a few TB cases, for example in patients with adverse reactions to rifampicin and/or pyrazinamide and new patients who refuse DOTS despite all efforts. This is a treatment regimen of 12-month duration comprising 2 months of SHE (streptomycin, isoniazid, ethambutol) and 10 months of HE (isoniazid, ethambutol) (2SHE/10HE).

Chemoprophylaxis or preventive chemotherapy with isoniazid is administered to all the children aged 6 years and below who are in contact with smear positive pulmonary TB cases.

The results of intermittent chemotherapy outcomes are shown in figures 9.1 and 9.2.

Since 1993, till 3rd quarter of 2009, over 35 lakh new smear positive patients were registered under RNTCP, and over 30 lakh patients (85%) have been successfully treated. Among smear positive retreatment cases, over 12 lakh patients were registered and the treatment success rate is over 70%. If one reduces default, which is 16%, the treatment success rate can be more than 80%, re-emphasizing that category II regimen is effective; however, the major challenge was the high default rate, which is around 16%. In any case, these are now categorized as MDR-TB suspects.

However, following World Health Organization recommendations and expert comments, the program is now changing into the daily therapy, which is being pilot tested in five states.

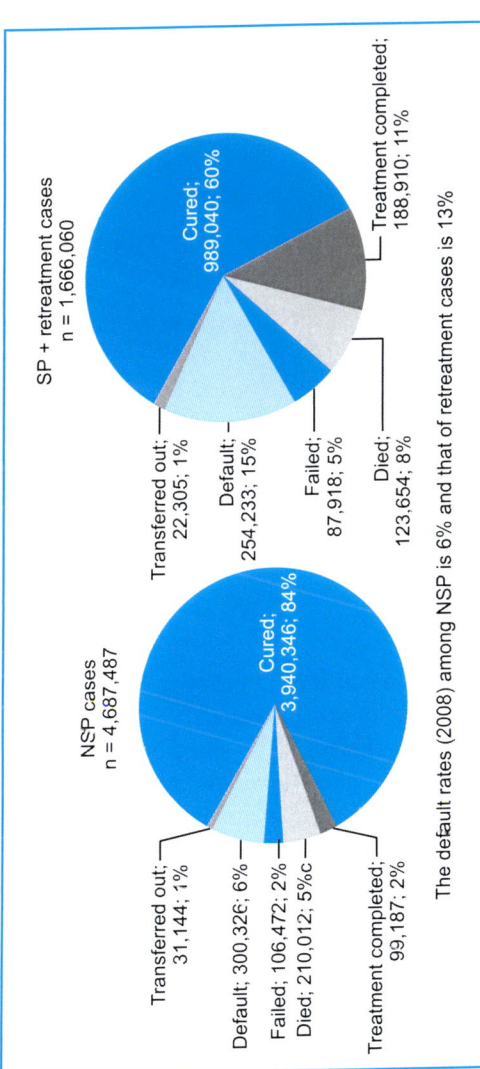

NSP, new smear positive; SP, smear positive.

Figure 9.1 Treatment outcome of smear positive cases (new and retreatment) registered under Revised National Tuberculosis Control Program directly observed treatment, short-course (1993–3Q2009).

Clinic Consult Pulmonology: Tuberculosis

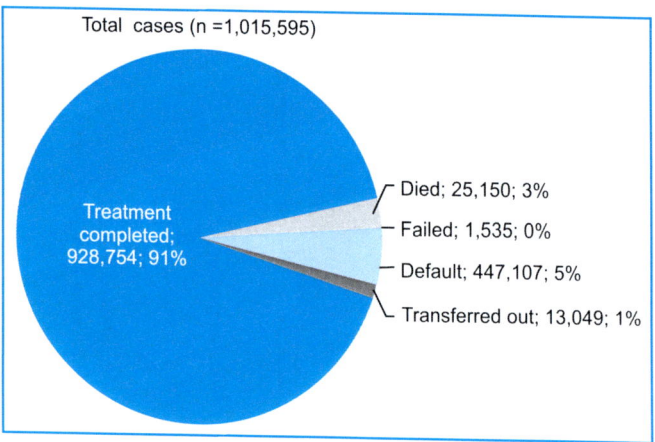

Figure 9.2: Treatment outcomes for new extrapulmonary tuberculosis (all forms) patients registered under Revised National Tuberculosis Control Program directly observed treatment, short-course (2005-3Q2009).

Side Effects

Most TB patients complete their treatment without any significant adverse drug effects. However, a few patients do experience adverse effects. It is, therefore, important that patients be clinically monitored during treatment so that adverse effects can be detected promptly and managed properly. Routine laboratory monitoring is not necessary.

Some drug-induced side effects like isoniazid-induced peripheral neuropathy can be prevented by health care professionals like DOT providers or the medical officer. This usually presents as numbness or a tingling or burning sensation of the hands or feet and occurs more commonly in pregnant women and in people with HIV infection, alcohol dependency, malnutrition, diabetes, chronic liver disease, and renal failure. These patients should receive preventive treatment with pyridoxine, 10 mg/day along with their anti-TB drugs (some guidelines recommend 25 mg/day).

In general, a patient who develops minor adverse effects should continue the TB treatment and be given symptomatic treatment. If a patient develops a major side effect, the treatment or the responsible drug is stopped; the patient should be urgently referred to a clinician or health care facility for further assessment and treatment. Patients with major adverse reactions should be managed in a hospital.

If a patient develops itching without a rash and there is no other obvious cause, the recommended approach is to try symptomatic treatment with antihistamines and skin moisturizing, and continue TB treatment while observing the patient closely. If a skin rash develops, however, all anti-TB drugs must be stopped. Once the reaction has resolved, anti-TB drugs are reintroduced one by one, starting with the drug least likely to be responsible for the reaction (rifampicin or isoniazid) at a small challenge dose, such as 50 mg isoniazid. The dose is gradually increased over 3 days. This procedure is repeated, adding in one drug at a time. A reaction after adding in a particular drug identifies that drug as the one responsible for the reaction. The alternative can be used when a particular drug cannot be used because it was implicated as the cause of a cutaneous reaction.

Isoniazid, pyrazinamide, and rifampicin can all cause liver damage (drug-induced hepatitis). In addition, rifampicin can cause asymptomatic jaundice without evidence of hepatitis. It is important to try to rule out other possible causes like viral hepatitis, alcoholic hepatitis, etc., before deciding that the hepatitis is induced by the TB regimen.

The management of hepatitis induced by TB treatment depends on:
- Whether the patient is in the intensive or continuation phase of TB treatment

- The severity of the liver disease
- The severity of the TB
- The capacity of the health unit to manage the side effects of TB treatment.

If the liver disease is caused by the anti-TB drugs, all drugs should be stopped. If the patient is severely ill with TB and it is considered unsafe to stop TB treatment, a nonhepatotoxic regimen consisting of streptomycin, ethambutol, and a fluoroquinolone should be started.

If TB treatment has been stopped, it is necessary to wait for liver function tests to revert to normal and clinical symptoms (nausea, abdominal pain) to resolve before reintroducing the anti-TB drugs. If it is not possible to perform liver function tests, it is advisable to wait an extra 2 weeks after resolution of jaundice and upper abdominal tenderness before restarting TB treatment. If the signs and symptoms do not resolve and the liver disease is severe, the nonhepatotoxic regimen consisting of streptomycin, ethambutol, and a fluoroquinolone should be started (or continued) for a total of 18–24 months.

Once drug-induced hepatitis has resolved, the drugs are reintroduced one at a time. If symptoms recur or liver function tests become abnormal as the drugs are reintroduced, the last drug added should be stopped. Some advice starting with rifampicin because it is less likely than isoniazid or pyrazinamide to cause hepatotoxicity and is the most effective agent. After 3–7 days, isoniazid may be reintroduced. In patients who have experienced jaundice but tolerate the reintroduction of rifampicin and isoniazid, it is advisable to avoid pyrazinamide. Alternative regimens depend on which drug is implicated as the cause of the hepatitis. If rifampicin is implicated, a suggested regimen without rifampicin is 2 months of isoniazid, ethambutol, and streptomycin followed by 10 months of isoniazid and ethambutol. If isoniazid cannot be used, 6–9 months of rifampicin, pyrazinamide, and ethambutol can be considered. If pyrazinamide is discontinued before the patient has completed the intensive phase, the total duration of isoniazid and rifampicin therapy may be extended to 9 months.

If neither isoniazid nor rifampicin can be used, the non-hepatotoxic regimen consisting of streptomycin, ethambutol, and a fluoroquinolone should be continued for a total of 18–24 months.

Reintroducing one drug at a time is the optimal approach, especially if the patient's hepatitis was severe. National TB control programs using fixed dose combination tablets should therefore, stock limited quantities of single anti-TB drugs for use in such cases. However, if the country's health units do not yet have single anti-TB drugs, clinical experience in resource-limited settings has been successful with the following approach, which depends on whether the hepatitis with jaundice occurred during the intensive or the continuation phase.

- When hepatitis with jaundice occurs during the intensive phase of TB treatment with isoniazid, rifampicin, pyrazinamide, and ethambutol: once hepatitis has resolved, restart the same drugs except replace pyrazinamide with streptomycin to complete the 2-month course of initial therapy, followed by rifampicin and isoniazid for the 6-month continuation phase
- When hepatitis with jaundice occurs during the continuation phase: once hepatitis has resolved, restart isoniazid and rifampicin to complete the 4-month continuation phase of therapy. Side-effects of various anti-tubercular drugs are shown in Table 9.7.

TABLE 9.7

Symptom-based approach to manage side effects of antituberculosis drugs

Side effects	Drug(s) probably responsible	Management
Major		Stop responsible drug(s) and refer to clinician urgently
Skin rash with or without itching	Streptomycin, isoniazid, rifampicin, pyrazinamide	Stop anti-TB drugs
Deafness (no wax on otoscopy)	Streptomycin	Stop streptomycin
Dizziness (vertigo and nystagmus)	Streptomycin	Stop streptomycin
Jaundice (other causes excluded), hepatitis	Isoniazid, pyrazinamide, rifampicin	Stop anti-TB drugs
Confusion (suspect drug-induced acute liver failure if there is jaundice)	Most anti-TB drugs	Stop anti-TB drugs
Visual impairment (other causes excluded)	Ethambutol	Stop ethambutol
Decreased urine output	Streptomycin	Stop streptomycin

Continued

Antituberculosis Drugs

Continued

Symptom-based approach to manage side effects of antituberculosis drugs

Side effects	Drug(s) probably responsible	Management
Minor		Continue anti-TB drugs, check drug doses
Anorexia, nausea, abdominal pain	Pyrazinamide, rifampicin, isoniazid	Give drugs with small meals or just before bedtime, and advice patient to swallow pills slowly with small sips of water. If symptoms persist or worsen, or there is protracted vomiting or any sign of bleeding, consider the side effect to be major and refer to clinician urgently
Joint pains	Pyrazinamide	Aspirin or nonsteroidal anti-inflammatory drug, or paracetamol
Burning, numbness, or tingling sensation in the hands or feet	Isoniazid	Pyridoxine 50–75 mg daily
Drowsiness	Isoniazid	Reassurance. Give drugs before bedtime
Orange/red urine	Rifampicin	Reassurance. Patients should be told when starting treatment that this may happen and is normal
Flu like syndrome (fever, chills, malaise, headache, bone pain)	Intermittent dosing of rifampicin	Change from intermittent to daily rifampicin administration

TB, tuberculosis.

PROPHYLAXIS

- Latent TB infection (LTBI) is defined as a state of persistent immune response to stimulation by *M. tuberculosis* antigens without evidence of clinically manifested active TB
- A direct measurement tool for *M. tuberculosis* infection in humans is currently unavailable
- Tuberculin skin test (TST) and interferon-γ release assays (IGRA) are indicative of infection but not disease. The vast majority of infected persons have no signs or symptoms of TB but are at risk for developing active TB disease
- One-third of the world's population is estimated to be infected with *M. tuberculosis*
- The lifetime risk of reactivation TB for a person with documented LTBI is estimated to be 5–10%, with the majority developing TB disease within the first 5 years after initial infection. However, the risk of developing TB disease following infection depends on several factors, the most important one being the immunological status of the host
- Reactivation TB can be averted by preventive treatment
- Currently available treatments have an efficacy ranging from 60 to 90%
- The potential benefit of treatment needs to be carefully balanced against the risk of drug related adverse events.

IDENTIFICATION OF HIGH RISK GROUP

In High-income and Upper Middle-income Countries with Estimated Tuberculosis Incidence Less than 100 per 100,000 Population

- Systematic testing and treatment of LTBI should be performed in people living with HIV, adult, and child

contacts of pulmonary TB cases, patients initiating anti-tumor necrosis factor treatment, patients receiving dialysis, patients preparing for organ or hematologic transplantation, and patients with silicosis. Either IGRA or Mantoux TST should be used to test for LTBI (strong recommendation, low to very low quality of evidence)
- Systematic testing and treatment of LTBI should be considered for prisoners, health workers, immigrants from high TB burden countries, homeless persons, and illicit drug users. Either IGRA or TST should be used to test for LTBI (conditional recommendation, low to very low quality of evidence)
- Systematic testing for LTBI is not recommended in people with diabetes, harmful alcohol use, tobacco smokers, and underweight people, unless they are already included in the above recommendations (conditional recommendation, very low quality of evidence)

For Resource-limited Countries and Other Middle-income Countries that Do Not Belong to the Above Category (According to Existing and Valid World Health Organization Guidelines)

- People living with HIV and children below 5 years of age who are household or close contacts of people with TB and who, after an appropriate clinical evaluation, are found not to have active TB but have LTBI should be treated (strong recommendation, high quality of evidence).

Remarks

Testing and treatment of LTBI should adhere to strict human rights and the highest ethical considerations. For example, positive test results or status of treatment for LTBI should

Clinic Consult Pulmonology: Tuberculosis

not affect a person's immigration status or delay the ability to immigrate. For people living with HIV and child contacts below 5 years of age, the existing WHO guidelines should be consulted.

- Individuals should be asked about symptoms of TB before being tested for LTBI. Chest radiography can be done if efforts are intended also for active TB case finding. Individuals with TB symptoms or any radiological abnormality should be investigated further for active TB and other conditions (strong recommendation, very low quality of evidence)
- Either TST or IGRA can be used to test for LTBI in high-income and upper middle-income countries with estimated TB incidence less than 100 per 100,000 (strong recommendation, very low quality of evidence)
- Interferon-γ release assays should not replace TST in low-income and other middle-income countries (strong recommendation, very low quality of evidence).
- HIV should be incorporated into the medical evaluation of LTBI treatment candidates based on national or local policies.

Treatment Options for Latent Tuberculosis Infection

The following treatment options are recommended for the treatment of LTBI (Table 9.8):

- 6-month isoniazid, or
- 9-month isoniazid, or
- 3-month regimen of weekly rifapentine plus isoniazid, or
- 3–4 months isoniazid plus rifampicin, or
- 3–4 months rifampicin alone.

Strong recommendation, moderate to high quality of evidence.

Antituberculosis Drugs

TABLE 9.8

Recommended drug usage		
Drug regimen	*Dose per body weight*	Maximum dose
Daily isoniazid alone for 6 or 9 months	• Adults = 5 mg/kg • Children = 10 mg/kg	• 300 mg
Daily rifampicin alone for 3–4 months	• Adults = 10 mg/kg • Children = 10 mg/kg	• 600 mg
Daily isoniazid plus rifampicin for 3–4 months	• *Isoniazid* • Adults = 5 mg/kg • Children = 10 mg/kg • *Rifampicin* • Adults and children = 10 mg/kg	• Isoniazid = 300 mg • Rifampicin = 600 mg
Weekly rifampenitine plus isoniazid for 3 months (12 doses)	• Adults and children • Isoniazid 15 mg/kg • Rifampenitine (by body weight) • 10.0–14.0 kg = 300 mg • 14.1–25.0 kg = 450 mg • 25.1–32.0 kg = 600 mg • 32.1–49.9 kg = 750 mg	• Isoniazid = 900 mg • Rifampicin = 600 mg

Remark

There was consensus of the panel on the equivalence of 6-month isoniazid, 9-month isoniazid, and 3-month rifapentine plus isoniazid. However, the panel could not reach a consensus and voted on the equivalence of 3–4 months isoniazid plus rifampicin and 3–4 months rifampicin alone as alternative options to 6-month isoniazid. Sixty percent of the panel members voted for 4-month rifampicin alone as an equivalent option to 6-month isoniazid, while 53% voted for 3–4 months isoniazid plus rifampicin as an equivalent option to 6-month isoniazid. Rifampicin and rifapentine containing regimens should be prescribed with caution to people living with HIV who are on antiretroviral treatment due to potential drug-to-drug interactions.

VACCINES

- Development of an efficacious vaccine against human TB remains a challenging goal despite a number of candidate vaccines are being tested and are in various stages of clinical development.
- New paradigms for research and development call for increased emphasis on experimental medicine, biomarker discovery, and novel clinical proof of concept studies to streamline vaccine development and maximize the probability of success in late-stage trials
- Emerging platforms and techniques for more effective delivery offer hope in paving the way for achieving the ultimate goal of breaking the infection-transmission-disease cycle, in an effort to substantially reduce the global burden of disease
- Till that time, Bacille Calmette-Guérin (BCG) vaccination remains the standard of vaccination against TB
- Bacille Calmette-Guérin was first used to immunize humans in 1921. It was introduced into the WHO expanded program on immunization in 1974. The global BCG vaccination coverage rates exceed 80% in many countries endemic for TB. Extensive clinical trials have been conducted to assess the protective efficacy of BCG against pulmonary TB, but a wide range of vaccine efficacy values have been observed. This is possibly due to differences in study design, geographical location, and presence and absence of nontuberculous mycobacteria. The greatest disadvantage of BCG vaccination is that it does not prevent reactivation of latent TB, which is the main source of bacillary dissemination in the community.

Despite these limitations, and particularly in light of the growing HIV/acquired immune deficiency syndrome pandemic and the appearance of multidrug-resistant *M. tuberculosis* strains, BCG vaccines will continue to represent an important tool in the global fight against TB until new vaccines are available for clinical use. In India, BCG vaccination is covered under the universal expanded program of immunization where in it is administered at birth till the age of 1 month. The only benefit is that it prevents the development of dissemination and tubercular meningitis

- *Mycobacterium indicus pranii* (MIP) and *M. vaccae* are in phase III clinical trial and the Drug Controller of India licensed MIP for human use in India.

KEY MESSAGE

❑ A number of anti-tuberculosis drugs are available, although development of newer drugs took a long time. The time-tested 5 important drugs are discussed in detail. The Revised National Tuberculosis Control Program of India as well as the WHO has recommended the use of combination chemotherapy whether the patient is new or has received treatment earlier. Drug resistance is a challenge. The RNTCP of India still uses the intermittent short course chemotherapy, but now changing to daily therapy very soon.

SUGGESTED READINGS

1. American Thoracic Society, CDC, Infectious Diseases Society of America. Treatment of tuberculosis. MMWR Morb Mortal Wkly Rep. 2003;52(RR-11):1-77.
2. da Costa C, Walker B, Bonavia A. Tuberculosis vaccines--state of the art, and novel approaches to vaccine development. Int J Infect Dis. 2015;32:5-12.

3. Guidelines for intensified tuberculosis case-finding and isoniazid preventive therapy for people living with HIV in resource-constrained settings. Geneva: World Health Organization; 2011.
4. Guidelines on the management of latent tuberculosis infection. World Health Organization; 2015.
5. Lobue P, Menzies D. Treatment of latent tuberculosis infection: an update. Respirology. 2010;15:603-22.
6. Ma Z, Lienhardt C, McIlleron H, Nunn AJ, Wang X. Global tuberculosis drug development pipeline: the need and the reality. Lancet. 2010;12;375:2100-9.
7. Recommendations for investigating contacts of persons with infectious tuberculosis in low- and middle income countries. Geneva: World Health Organization; 2012.
8. Roy A, Eisenhut M, Harris RJ, Rodrigues LC, Sridhar S, Habermann S, et al. Effect of BCG vaccination against Mycobacterium tuberculosis infection in children: systematic review and meta-analysis. BMJ. 2014;349:g4643.
9. Saukkonen JJ, , Cohn DL, Jasmer RM, Schenker S, Jereb JA, Nolan CM, et al. An official ATS statement: hepatotoxicity of antituberculosis therapy. Am J Respir Crit Care Med. 2006;174:935-52.
10. Toman K. Toman's tuberculosis. Case detection, treatment, and monitoring: questions and answers. 2nd ed. Geneva: World Health Organization; 2004.
11. Treatment of tuberculosis Guidelines. 4th ed. WHO/HTM/TB/2009.420. World Health Organization; 2010.
12. WHO Model Formulary 2008. Geneva: World Health Organization; 2009. Available from: www.who.int/selection_medicines/list/WMF 2008.pdf.
13. Williams G, Alarcon E, Jittimanee S, Walusimbi M, Sebek M, Berga E, et al. Best practice of the care for patients with tuberculosis: a guide for low income countries. International Union against Tuberculosis and Lung Disease, Paris; 2007.
14. Williams G, Alarcon E, Jittimanee S, Walusimbi M, Sebek M, Berga E, et al. Care during the intensive phase: promotion of adherence. Int J Tuberc Lung Dis. 2008;12:601-5.

CHAPTER 10
Revised National Tuberculosis Control Program of India

INTRODUCTION

The Revised National Tuberculosis Control Program (RNTCP) has published the new Technical and Operational Guidelines in 2016 for tuberculosis (TB) control in India. They are discussed in brief in this chapter. These guidelines can be practiced by all physicians at all levels.

CASE FINDING AND EARLY DIAGNOSIS

Early case detection is important for early cure and prevention of transmission in the society. Case finding is also important to achieve 90% case detection and reporting as planned in the National Strategic Plan. Earlier approach of passive case detection leaves out a large number of cases besides delayed diagnosis. Therefore, presumptive cases of TB should be tested for presence of TB. Enhanced outreach attempts and screening at each point of contact with the healthcare should be the strategy.

Tuberculosis Suspect (Presumptive Pulmonary Tuberculosis)

Any of the symptoms or signs suggestive of TB including:

- Cough more than 2 weeks
- Fever more than 2 weeks
- Significant weight loss
- Hemoptysis
- Abnormality in chest skiagram.

In addition, these groups should be regularly screened for symptoms and signs of TB:
- Contacts of microbiologically confirmed TB cases
- People living with human immunodeficiency virus (PLHIV)
- Diabetes mellitus
- Cancer patients
- Malnourished
- Patients with immunosuppressive or steroids
- Homeless persons, prisons, destitute.

Presumptive Extrapulmonary Tuberculosis

Presence of organ specific symptoms or signs like:
- Lymph node swelling
- Joint pain and swelling
- Neck stiffness, disorientation, and/or
- Constitutional symptoms like significant weight loss, persistent fever for more than or equal to 2 weeks, night sweats, etc.

Presumptive Pediatric Tuberculosis

- Persistent fever and or cough more than 2 weeks
- Loss of weight (history of unexplained weight loss or no weight gain, in past 3 months; loss of weight is defined as loss of more than 5% of body weight compared to highest weight recorded in the last 3 months)/no weight gain, and/or
- History of contact with infectious TB cases (in a symptomatic child, contact with any form of active TB within last 2 years).

Presumptive Drug-resistant Tuberculosis

- Those patients who have failed treatment with first line drugs
- Pediatric TB nonresponders
- Drug-resistant (DR)-TB or rifampicin-resistant TB contacts
- Tuberculosis patients positive sputum on any follow-up sputum examination during treatment with first line drugs
- Previously treated TB cases
- Tuberculopsis patients with HIV coinfection.

DIGNOSTIC METHODS UNDER REVISED NATIONAL TUBERCULOSIS CONTROL PROGRAM

All efforts should be made to confirm the diagnosis in a presumptive cases using appropriate biological samples. For pulmonary TB it is sputum and for extrapulmonary TB it is the tissue/fluid samples like pleural fluid or cerebrospinal fluid (CSF) and histological samples in appropriate cases.

Sputum Smear Microscopy (for Acid Fast Bacilli)

- Zeihl-Neelson (ZN) staining
- Fluorescence staining.

Culture

- Solid [Lowenstein Jensen (LJ)] media
- Automated liquid culture systems (BACTEC MGIT 960, BactiAlert, Versatrek, etc.)
- Drug susceptibility testing (DST)
- Modified PST for MGIT 960 system (for both first and second line drugs)
- Economic variants of proportion sensitivity testing (1%) using LJ medium (as back up when indicated).

Rapid Molecular Testing

- Line probe assay (LPA) for *M. tuberculosis* complex and detection of resistance to rifampicin and isoniazid
- Nucleic acid amplification test (NAAT)/X-pert MTB/RIF testing using Gene Xpert system.

Although less sensitive, sputum microscopy using ZN stain has been the cornerstone of TB diagnosis for several decades and the RNTCP. It is relatively cheap and could be done at all circumstances and situations and it is technically quite simple. The sensitivity is still low in children and in PLHIV. Under the RNTCP, two microscopic methods—the ZN staining using the conventional microscope and light emitting diode fluorescent based microscopy—are used. Two sputum samples are collected within a day or on two consecutive days.

Culture methods are highly sensitive and specific, but takes time for 2–8 weeks and hence cannot be used for early diagnosis. However, they are useful for detecting and following up of cases of DR-TB to detect any early recurrence or cure.

Nucleic acid amplification test provides accurate and rapid diagnosis of TB by detecting the organism and rifampicin resistance conferring mutations (rpoB gene) in sputum as well as specimens from extrapulmonary TB like CSF and lymph nodes. Presently, RNTCP only recommends the use of this GeneXpert for the diagnosis of DR-TB in presumptive DR-TB cases and TB preferentially in key populations like children, PLHIV and some extrapulmonary TB cases.

Other Diagnostic Tests

Radiography

Diagnosis of pulmonary TB by using chest radiographs may be unreliable as it is of low specificity although has a high sensitivity. Any abnormality in a TB suspect should further be evaluated microbiologically. In the absence of microbiological confirmation, the diagnosis of TB should be made very carefully taking into account other symptoms and signs. In that even the diagnosis is labeled as "clinically diagnosed TB".

Tuberculin Skin Test and Interferon Gamma Release Assays

Tuberculin skin test (TST) may be used in cases of children in combination with history of contact, symptoms, radiology, and microbiology. Interferon-γ release assays (IGRA) is being used instead of TST in low prevalence countries. In countries like India, its advantage over TST is uncertain and perhaps has no advantage, rather it adds to the cost of investigation. Both TST and IGRA are not recommended in the diagnostic algorithm of TB in adults.

Other Serological Tests

The Government of India has banned the manufacture, import, distribution, and use of currently available commercial serological tests for diagnosis of TB. Hence, they are not recommended for diagnosis of TB.

All TB suspects whether in the public sector or private sector should undergo the following algorithm as shown in figure 10.1.

TREATMENT OF TUBERCULOSIS

The goals of TB treatment are to decrease the case fatality and morbidities associated with untreated TB by ensuring cure that is to be relapse free, to minimize and prevent the development of drug resistance, and to make the patient noninfectious, which will break the chain of transmission in the society to other healthy individuals and to decrease the pool of infection.

Clinic Consult Pulmonology: Tuberculosis

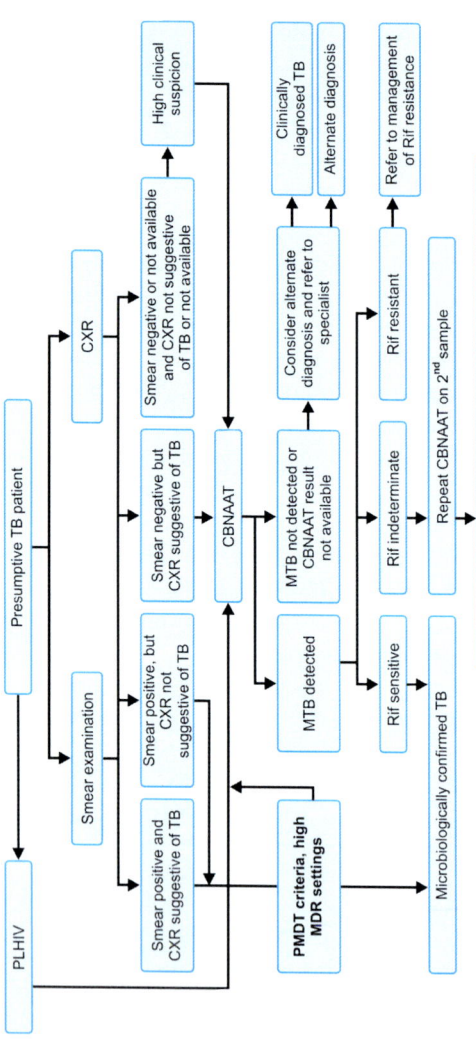

PLHIV, people living with human immunodeficiency virus; CXR, chest X-ray; TB, tuberculosis; PMDT, Programmatic Management of Drug-resistant TB; MDR, multidrug-resistant; MTB, Mycobacterium tuberculosis; CBNAAT, cartridge based nucleic acid amplification test; Rif, rifampicin; LPA, line probe assay.

Figure 10:1: Diagnostic algorithm for pulmonary tuberculosis (Revised National Tuberculosis Control Program of India, 2016).

Note: All presumptive TB cases should be offered HIV counseling and testing. However, diagnostic work-up for TB must not be delayed.

Case Definitions

A case of TB can either be any of the following.

Microbiologically Confirmed Case of Tuberculosis

This is a presumptive case of TB patient in whom a biological sample/specimen is positive for acid-fast bacilli, positive on culture, or positive through quality assured rapid diagnostic molecular test.

They can further be classified according to:
- Anatomical site of the disease
- History of previous treatment
- Drug resistance.

Note

- If the first smear is positive and if the patient is not at risk for drug-resistant tuberculosis (DR-TB), he/she will be categorized as "microbiologically confirmed TB (sensitivity status not known)"
- Smear positive and presumptive multidrug resistant-TB (MDR-TB) as per Programmatic. Management of Drug Resistant TB guidelines, and in settings of high MDR-TB (MDR-TB rates >5% among new cases and >20% among retreatment cases), a cartridge based nucleic acid amplification test (CBNAAT; GeneXpert) will be performed to rule out rifampicin resistance before initiation of treatment and the patient will be categorized as "microbiologically confirmed drug sensitive TB (DST)" or "rifampicin-resistant TB"
- If the first smear is negative, chest X-ray may be considered and if suggestive of TB, the second sample will be subjected to smear and CBNAAT simultaneously

Clinic Consult Pulmonology: Tuberculosis

- Based on CBNAAT results, the patient will be categorized as "microbiologically confirmed drug sensitive TB (DST)" or "rifampicin-resistance TB". If negative, other differential diagnosis is to be considered
- Rifampicin indeterminate result will be tested for another CBNAAT to get a valid result. In the event of indeterminate result again on the second occasion also, an additional specimen will be collected and will be sent to the nearest Intermediate reference laboratory or culture and drug susceptibility testing (C and DST) center for line probe assays or liquid culture and DST as appropriate
- Subject to availability of a suitable accredited laboratory efforts should be made to obtain DST results by collecting additional samples
- If both the sputum smear and chest X-ray are negative, and the physician is still suspecting TB, the patient must be referred to a pulmonary/chest specialist
- All key population like people living with human immunodeficiency virus, children, and extrapulmonary TB should get an upfront CBNAAT
- All the healthcare diagnostic facilities should be quality assured by competent health authorities.

Classification based on anatomical site of the disease:

1. Pulmonary TB: Any microbiologically confirmed or clinically diagnosed case of TB involving the lung parenchyma or the tracheobronchial tree.
2. Extrapulmonary TB: Any microbiologically confirmed or clinically diagnosed case of TB involving organs other than lungs like pleura, lymph nodes, meninges, central nervous system, bones and joints, urogenital system, gastrointestinal system, pericardium, and skin.

Miliary TB is classified as pulmonary TB as the lungs are involved. A case of both pulmonary TB and extrapulmonary TB is classified as a case of pulmonary TB.

Classification based on history of treatment of tuberculosis:
1. New case of TB: A patient who has never taken anti-TB treatment or if taken the drugs, the duration was less than 1 month.
2. Previously treated case: The patient has taken treatment with anti-TB drugs for more than a month in the past.
   a. Recurrent TB case: A patient previously declared as successfully treated (cured/treatment completed) and subsequently found to be microbiologically confirmed TB case.
   b. Treatment after failure: These are patients who have previously treated for TB and whose treatment failed at the end of their most recent course of treatment.
   c. Treatment after loss to follow-up: A TB patient previously treated for TB for 1 month or more and was declared lost to follow up in their recent course of treatment and subsequently found microbiologically confirmed TB case.
   d Other previously treated patients: These patients have previously been treated for TB but whose outcome after their most recent course of treatment in unknown or undocumented.
3. Transferred in: A TB patient who has received treatment in a TB unit, after registered for treatment in another TB unit is considered as a case of transferred in.

Tuberculosis is also classified according to drug resistance as monoresistant TB, polydrug-resistant TB, multidrug-resistant TB, rifampicin-resistant TB, and extensive DR-TB.

Clinically Diagnosed Case of Tuberculosis

This is a presumptive case of TB patient who is not confirmed microbiologically or by molecular testing but has been diagnosed clinically by a clinician on the basis of a chest radiograph, histopathology, or clinical signs with a decision to treat the patient with a full-course of anti-TB drugs.

In children, the clinical diagnosis is based on abnormalities consistent with TB on chest X-ray, a history of contact with a infectious case, evidence of infection with TB (positive Mantoux test), and clinical findings suggestive of TB in children in the event of negative or unavailable microbiological tests.

DRUG REGIMEN

Treatment for Drug Sensitive Tuberculosis

The RNTCP follows thrice weekly regimen as discussed earlier for drug sensitive and retreatment cases (categories I and II cases). The program, however, is now advocating/introducing daily regimen for drug sensitive TB among PLHIV and pediatric TB patients throughout the country and for all TB patients in 104 districts of 5 states—Himachal Pradesh, Sikkim, Bihar, Maharashtra, and Kerala—covering a population of 2,690 lakhs. The remaining states will continue with the intermittent regimen as per existing guidelines until the daily regimen is scaled up to the entire country after a pilot testing in the above 5 states.

The principle of daily treatment regimen (other than drug resistant cases) is to administer daily fixed dose combinations of first line anti-TB drugs according to the four weight bands. The drug regimen is shown in table 10.1.

TABLE 10.1

Daily drug regimens for tuberculosis cases as recommended by Revised National Tuberculosis Control Program		
Type of TB case	Treatment regimen in IP	Treatment regimen CP
New	(2) HRZE	(4) HRE
Previously treated	(2) HRZES + (1) HRZE	(5) HRE

IP, intensive phase; CP, continuation phase; H, isoniazid; R, rifampin; Z, pyrazinamide; E, ethambutol; S, streptomycin.

Note: Prefix to the drugs stands for numger of months.

For new cases of TB, the treatment in the intensive phase (IP) consists of 8 weeks of isoniazid, rifampicin, pyrazinamide, and ethambutol in daily doses as per weight band categories. There will be no need for extension of IP. Pyrazinamide is stopped in the continuatiuon phase (CP), while the other three drugs are continued for another 16 weeks as daily doses completing a total of 24 weeks.

For previously treated cases of TB, the IP will be of 12 weeks, where injection streptomycin is added for first 2 months (8 weeks) along with the other four drugs and the injection is stopped for the next 4 weeks of the 12 weeks of IP when the other four drugs are continued for another 4 weeks. During the next 20 weeks, three drugs are continued and pyrazinamide is discontinued during this period. All drugs are used daily in both the phases for a total of 32 weeks.

The CP in both the new and previously treated cases may be extended for another 12–24 weeks in certain forms of TB like central nervous system TB, skeletal TB, disseminated TB, etc. based on the clinical decision of the treating physician. Extension beyond 12 weeks should only be on the recommendation of experts of the concerned field.

Loose drugs would be required as substitutes in cases of adverse drug reactions or with comorbid conditions.

Clinic Consult Pulmonology: Tuberculosis

> **KEY MESSAGE**
>
> ❑ The Revised National Tuberculosis Control Program of India has recently updated the guidelines for the diagnosis and treatment of tuberculosis. The suspect criteria for TB been expanded. The program has now changed into the daily therapy regimen while earlier one was an intermittent therapy. This will be pilot tested initially. All practicing physicians dealing with tuberculosis should read and practice these guidelines.

SUGGESTED READING

1. Revised National tuberculosis Control Program. Technical and Operational Guidelines for tuberculosis control in India. 2016. Central TB Division, Directorate General of Health services, Ministry of Health and Family Welfare, Government of India, New Delhi.